The Chronic Pain Patient
Evaluation and Management

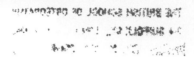

Pain and Headache

Vol. 7

Series Editor
Philip L. Gildenberg, Houston, Tex.

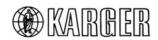

S. Karger · Basel · München · Paris · London · New York · Tokyo · Sydney

The Chronic Pain Patient

Evaluation and Management

Philip L. Gildenberg, MD, PhD

Clinical Professor of Neurosurgery, University of Texas Medical School at Houston, Houston, Tex.

Richard A. DeVaul, MD

Dean, College of Medicine, University of West Virginia, Morgantown, W. Va.

4 tables, 1985

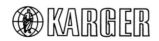

S. Karger · Basel · München · Paris · London · New York · Tokyo · Sydney

Pain and Headache

National Library of Medicine, Cataloging in Publication
   Gildenberg, Philip Leon, 1935 –
   The chronic pain patient: evaluation and management
   Philip L. Gildenberg, Richard A. DeVaul. – Basel; New York: Karger, 1985.
   (Pain and headache; v. 7)
   Includes index.
   1. Chronic Disease   2. Chronic Disease – therapy   3. Pain   4. Pain – therapy
   I. DeVaul, Richard A.   II. Title   III. Series
   Wl PA293 v.7 [WL 704 G468c]
   ISBN 3–8055–3911–8

Drug Dosage
   The authors and the publisher have exerted every effort to ensure that drug selection and dosage
   set forth in this text are in accord with current recommendations and practice at the time of
   publication. However, in view of ongoing research, changes in government regulations, and the
   constant flow of information relating to drug therapy and drug reactions, the reader is urged to
   check the package insert for each drug for any change in indications and dosage and for added
   warnings and precautions. This is particularly important when the recommended agent is a new
   and/or infrequently employed drug.

Contents

Contents

Acknowledgement

The authors wish to acknowledge with appreciation and respect the significant contributions of our editorial associates, *Patricia O. Franklin* and *Faith Jervy,* without whose participation this volume would not have been possible. Not only did they help us formulate our ideas into a manageable format, help assure that the manner of presentation was comprehensible, and were instrumental in making the transition from thought to paper, but they provided the impetus to bring the project to completion.

Philip L. Gildenberg
Richard A. DeVaul

Introduction

This volume describes a practical approach to the patient with chronic pain complaints, who has no identifiable *illness* amenable to medical treatment or structural pathology requiring surgery. This problem is frequent, frustrating, and particularly likely to lead to mismanagement and perpetuation of the patient's problems. After years of experience, the authors believe that most physicians are poorly prepared to recognize, understand and confront the central issues involved in a successful intervention with these patients.

Several dilemmas are involved. The patient presents with persistent pain and the urgency usually associated with acute illness, while the major problem is related to disability secondary to prolonged patienthood. Physicians are primarily trained in acute medical interventions and generally operate under the principle of identifying organic or treatable illness. In addition, insurance companies, the legal profession and employers view the patient as either completely sick and disabled or capable of full function. There is little social support for patients who need to recover and rehabilitate. We believe that this volume offers a step-by-step approach to patients with chronic pain when the central issue is not care by the doctor, but rehabilitation by the patient.

The program outlined here was developed at our Chronic Pain Clinic at The University of Texas Medical School at Houston. For 8 years we evaluated approximately 125 patients per year, and two-thirds of them took part in a 3-week inpatient program. The vast majority of patients had significant improvement in managing their pain and, more importantly, a marked lessening in their social disability with improvement in personal functioning. Some patients refused to accept the recommendations inherent in this approach. Some of these patients had too great a psychological or financial investment in their sick role to accept rehabilitation. Even for these patients the physician using this approach avoids adding to the patient's problems by offering harmful medications and possibly lessens the patient's current problem of chronic patienthood. Eventually, a number of patients who initially refused this approach saw its merit upon reflection and returned to become involved in a real rehabilitation program.

We saw patients only by referral from a physician. Ordinarily, the patients had already been under the care of physicians for months prior to their visit to us, yet many of the techniques we use could be employed by the primary physician and many of the concepts that form the basis for these techniques could also be used to formulate programs to prevent patients from becoming chronic pain patients.

Consequently, it seemed appropriate to present the philosophy and details of our program to other physicians. It is hoped that many patients with chronic pain will be successfully cared for without having to be referred to one of the growing number of comprehensive chronic pain clinics, and, more importantly, that additional patients will avoid the misdirection that leads down the pathway to chronic pain.

The concepts outlined here are not original with us. Some ideas were taken from pain clinics that preceded ours. Many of the concepts evolved simultaneously in our practice and in other pain clinics with similar approaches.

Most of the comprehensive chronic pain centers have similar orientations. They recognize the *complete failure of analgesic medication to control chronic pain* as well as the dangers inherent in most of these medications. Most incorporate a protocol for treating regression and secondary depression with the use of antidepressant medications. Most involve psychiatrists and/or psychologists in counseling programs of varying types intended to break the attitude of chronic pain and chronic disability behavior. Most have programs of gradually increasing physical activity, and most employ certain specific techniques for the treatment of pain per se, but only in the context of a comprehensive program. The details vary from one clinic to another, and yet their success rates appear to be similar. Consequently, we do not pretend the program we outline here is the only answer to chronic pain, but we allege that it is necessary to involve the patient in a multi-faceted comprehensive program in order to optimize the chances for success.

The objectives of this book are threefold. First, we want to acquaint the primary care physician with the identifying characteristics of a chronic pain syndrome patient. Second, we detail guidelines for thorough physical and psychosocial evaluation of these patients, a very important part of which is close and careful history-taking. Third, we describe the comprehensive approach to management of the chronic pain patient. The primary care physician may feel that the patient could benefit from admission to a chronic pain unit or he may wish to undertake management himself. In the former case, the patient is usually referred back to the primary physician after his stay in the chronic pain unit, so it is always important for the referring physician to understand the treatment philosophy and to be able to continue to guide the patient's rehabilitation.

While a comprehensive review of the literature on pain is beyond the scope of this volume, a few additional readings are suggested at the end of most chapters.

Chapter I

What Is Pain?

It is sadly recognized that the word 'pain' has no standard definition. Pain is the most common symptom that brings a patient to the physician. Virtually every doctor in every specialty has had occasion to see a patient whose presenting complaint was pain. Why do some of these patients do well, while others return again and again to haunt the physician because their pain fails to respond to treatment? Why do some patients spend their entire lives wracked with pain? Why does pain become the most important thing in the lives of some patients, developing into the major focus of every waking minute?

In general, pain can be divided into three categories, *acute pain, chronic pain* and *pain of malignancy.* Each of these categories will be discussed, but the chief concern of the book will be chronic pain, not acute pain nor pain of cancer.

Because the word 'pain' is used in so many different ways, the use of the word may impair rather than improve communication. For example, at a multidisciplinary international conference on pain, a variety of scientists were represented. Neurophysiologists used the word 'pain' to mean the appropriate response of specific pathways within the nervous system to a noxious stimulus, that is, a stimulus with the potential for producing tissue injury. Experimental psychologists meant a behavioral response to such a stimulus; one which implied that the pain pathways were being stimulated. Neurologists meant that the patient perceived pain, either because appropriate noxious stimulus was applied or because the nervous system was not functioning properly. Clinical psychologists meant that an individual complained of pain, whether or not a physiologic stimulus was identified. Psychiatrists meant that a patient was in distress, which was expressed as a disagreeable somatic sensation. Acupuncturists meant a complaint of a disagreeable sensation which may or may not have been permanently alleviated by influencing a 'pain pathway'. Each group reported accurately what they saw, and yet violent arguments developed between groups. Each scientist spoke only to the members of his own group, since each group defined the word 'pain' differently, and no one included in his individual presentation his definition of the word 'pain'.

If objective scientists have so much difficulty communicating by using an ill-defined term such as 'pain', how difficult is it for a patient to convey the distress he feels to a physician? How easy is it for a physician to apply his own definition, even though the patient may mean something else? How easy is it for a physician to assume automatically that the complaint of pain is related to a specific physical illness and treat the patient inappropriately? How easy is it for a physician to write a prescription for an analgesic when the cause of the patient's pain is not immediately apparent?

The word pain is used to describe a subjective perception of distress. It is not a simple sensation like the primary sensations. It cannot be quantified, as can a thermal, visual or auditory sensation. It is not as consistent as proprioception or two-point discrimination. It is not as well defined as touch sensation. It is not interpreted as concretely as stereognosis or graphesthesia. It is attended by a greater emotional response than any of these. It is complex and subject to individual interpretation.

Because pain is purely subjective, it cannot be measured. The physician must rely solely on the patient's report and try to imagine what the patient perceives. Yet, there may be no apparent cause for the patient's complaint, or the degree of distress may be far in excess of what might be anticipated from the description of the pain. It must be stressed, however, that the patient's pain is just as real whether or not there is a physical cause. The patient is just as disabled if the pain is partly or wholly from psychological causes and may require just as much help.

In the final analysis, 'Pain is what hurts.'

Suggested Reading

1   DeVaul, R.A.; Zisook, S.; Lorimor, R.: Patients with chronic pain. Med. J. St. Joseph Hosp. (Houston) *12:* 59–63 (1977).
2   Sternbach, R.A.: Pain patients, traits and treatment (Academic Press, New York 1974).

Chapter II

Physiologic and Psychological Contributors to Pain

While we may be unable to define the subjective experience of pain, we can attempt to describe it by considering its sources, pathways of transmission and the physiologic and psychologic conditions which affect one's perception and tolerance of pain.

The terms *threshold* and *tolerance* are important to an understanding of pain perception and are often confused. *Threshold* refers to the intensity of the stimulus which is first perceived as being painful. Thus, if the skin is heated, subjects consistently report the stimulus as being painful at a temperature of about 45 °C. This represents the threshold at which those nerve fibers concerned with pain perception are activated. Not coincidentally, this represents the temperature at which tissue damage first begins to occur. Since 'hot' equals 'warm' plus 'pain', it represents the thermal equivalent of a painful stimulus.

If each of a group of subjects exposed an area of skin to a temperature above that threshold and were asked not to withdraw until they could bear it no longer, there would be a great variation in the responses. Some subjects would withdraw almost immediately. Others would persist to the point of frank tissue damage. The ability to maintain control over one's self despite pain is *pain tolerance*. It varies from individual to individual, varies with age, with cultural training, and more importantly, with emotional state. Individuals who are depressed, anxious or fatigued tolerate the pain less well. Indeed, their perception of pain appears to be heightened, so they report the stimulus as being more intense than it actually is. For example, one of the characteristics of the agitation associated with narcotic withdrawal is a decrease in pain tolerance.

Although we may not be able to affect the source of the painful stimulus in certain chronic conditions, very often we can help the patient to improve his pain tolerance, that is, enable him to cope with the pain better. In doing so, the perception of pain is actually diminished. If the patient can cope with the pain without undue anxiety or depression, the pain itself may become less.

This is not to be confused with the allegation that 'The pain is all in his head,' or simply, 'You must learn to cope with the pain.'

If the patient has underlying anxiety or depression, and especially if the pain intensifies those emotions, tolerance to the pain may decrease. This has the effect of heightening the pain perception, which increases the attendant anxiety and depression. This in turn decreases the tolerance, and so forth. A vicious cycle is set up, wherein the patient's emotional response to the pain may in itself make the pain worse. If this cycle is broken at several emotional as well as physical points, it is sometimes possible to decrease the patient's pain significantly without altering the source of the painful stimulus.

There is another psychophysical phenomenon which creates a vicious pain cycle. In patients who have pain attendant to muscle injury, particularly muscles of the trunk or neck, the injured muscle may go into local spasm and produce pain. It is recognized that patients who are anxious or tense have an unconscious reflex increase in muscle tension, most commonly in those muscles of the neck or trunk which support the body and the weight of the head. If those muscles are painful and already in spasm, further tension may increase the pain, and another vicious cycle is initiated. A muscle is injured and becomes spastic and consequently painful. The pain creates emotional tension and anxiety which create increased tension in the muscle, which in turn increases the pain. The increased pain further increases the emotional response and the vicious cycle perpetuates the pain. This effect is very often seen after flexion-extension injuries of the neck that occur after rear-end collisions or in chronic low back strain.

When one is confronted with a patient with pain, particularly one with chronic pain, it is helpful to consider that the pain may have *physiologic, pathologic* or *psychologic* components. The pain may represent any one of these separately, or may be a combination of two or even all three. Since both the evaluation and the management of these pain components are different, the patient may require either a simple or a comprehensive program.

Physiologic pain is that pain which results from the appropriate response of an intact nervous system to a noxious or tissue-destructive stimulus which may arise from pathology within the body. The pain-sensitive nerve endings in the tissue fire and the information is transmitted via the pain pathways to the brain. This sequence occurs in acute pain generated by the application of a noxious stimulus but may not occur at all in chronic pain. It is appropriate to feel pain when a bone is broken. It is appropriate to feel pain when there is an inflammatory condition. It is appropriate to feel pain on stepping on a nail. Physiologic pain is a basic protective sensation and is important to the survival of the species and of the individual. Unfortunately, when the noxious stimulus represents an injury that does not heal or a prolonged pathologic process, such as cancer, this naturally protective physiologic pain can in itself be distressing and disabling.

Pathologic pain, from the standpoint of this discussion, refers to pain that occurs from pathology of the nervous system, rather than pain which occurs from pathology elsewhere in the body. The pain pathways may be firing, even though no noxious stimulus is being applied. The transmission lines are faulty, so when a non-noxious stimulus is applied, the static garbles the message and the pain pathways fire inappropriately. This is the pain that occurs with peripheral neuropathy, where damage to peripheral nerves lowers their threshold so that pain nerves may fire spontaneously. This is the pain of causalgia or dysesthesia, in which pain nerves may fire even on the application of a non-noxious or touch stimulus. Attention is directed to treating the nervous system rather than the body. If that is not possible, one may have to be satisfied with helping the patient to cope with the pain or using one of the specific therapies discussed later.

In *psychologic pain,* pain tolerance is poor, so that even moderately disagreeable sensations may be perceived as pain. The patient may be in an emotional state such as depression, wherein sensations ordinarily not painful are misinterpreted or improperly perceived as being painful. No stimulus may be applied, the pain pathways are not firing, but pain is perceived because of psychologic distress. In a state such as hysteria or conversion pain, there may be no somatic component to the pain at all, but the patient perceives pain.

In examining the patient with chronic pain, it is helpful to keep the three 'P's' of pain in mind and to attempt to weigh *how much of each component is present.* How much of the pain is from physiologic, pathologic, or psychologic factors? Does a pathologic condition such as malignancy or prolonged muscle spasm exist to cause the pain? Is there malfunction of the nervous system, such as a radiculopathy or peripheral neuropathy which may be exciting the pain pathways? Even in the presence of a somatic etiology, how much of the pain is a function of psychological cause, such as anxiety or depression? Is the patient's pain tolerance affected by these conditions or by narcotic withdrawal, so that perception of pain is heightened and tolerance to pain decreased, thereby initiating one of the vicious cycles discussed above?

Several other distinctions can be made between kinds and sources of pain, and making such distinctions enables us to describe the pain experience more accurately. For example, *acute pain* may be further subdivided into *fast pain* and *slow pain*. When a painful or noxious stimulus is suddenly applied, a sharp, well-localized, discrete fast pain is felt immediately and lasts momentarily. This is soon followed by a sensation of slow pain, a duller, aching, more diffuse and poorly localized disagreeable sensation. Think of the last time you stepped on a nail. The first perception was an acute lancinating pain that caused you to withdraw your foot. It was sharp and sharply localized. This was followed a few seconds later by an aching or burning sensation which involved not only the point of contact with the nail, but perhaps the entire foot. This persistent slow pain may be more distressing than the initial fast pain that preceded it. The fast pain is the result of a sudden transmission along the direct rapidly conducting nerve pathways. The slow pain may be mediated by a locally liberated chemical substance, may be transmitted by slowly conducting multisynaptic pathways, and may persist long after the cause is gone. This physiological distinction has nothing to do with speed of conduction of the nerves which perceive pain or with the distinction between acute and chronic pain, although the physiologic component of chronic pain may be of the slow variety.

One may hear acute pain designated as *somatic* or *visceral*. Somatic pain generally emanates from the musculoskeletal system, is well-localized and discrete. Visceral pain ordinarily emanates from the viscera within the body cavity, is poorly localized, aching or cramping in nature, and may have a large autonomic response associated with it. Although these classifications are helpful in evaluating acute pain, they are not often of assistance in analyzing chronic pain, since most chronic pain tends to be aching in nature and relatively diffuse.

Awareness of the concept of *referred pain* is important. Pain that emanates from a given location in the body may be perceived by the patient as being located somewhere else, usually in the same dermatome or an area supplied by the same peripheral nerve. The most common example of referred pain involves the myofascial syndrome from injury to muscle in the lumbosacral area, which may include pain that travels down the leg, even in the absence of a herniated disc or traumatized nerve root. The referred nature of the pain is suggested if the leg pain disappears on local anesthetic blocks of a trigger point in the lumbosacral area. Thus, a search for the origin of the pain in the leg or in the nerve root would be fruitless, whereas treatment of the lumbosacral area may alleviate the leg as well as the back pain.

This is not to be confused with *projected pain,* which results when pain of neuropathic origin is perceived along the distribution of the nerve. Thus, a herniated disc pressing on a lumbar or sacral nerve root in the back may be perceived as pain radiating down the leg. In projected pain, however, the pathology involves the nerve or nerve root itself, whereas in referred pain the pathology involves some other body tissue innervated by the same dermatome or nerve as the area of perceived pain.

No discussion of the physiology of pain is complete without mention of the *gate theory* of *Melzack and Wall.* They introduced the concept in 1965 in an attempt to reconcile a number of observations on the perception of pain with facts and theories about the physiology of the manner in which the pain pathways interpreted a stimulus as being painful. They elucidated the interrelationship of the several sensory nerves converging through the dorsal horn of the spinal cord in the substantia gelatinosa.

Although the concepts originally introduced by *Melzack and Wall* have proved to be incomplete and, in some regards, not in agreement with subsequent information, the concept remains valid and has served as a basis for certain pain treatments that will be discussed later.

The gate theory can be stated simply as, 'If you rub it, it feels better.'

Disregarding for a moment the technical details of the relationship of those nerves, we can summarize the theory by saying that whether or not pain is perceived depends on the balance between non-noxious and noxious stimuli. Stimulation that is not painful causes the large nerve fibers to fire. Noxious stimulation fires the higher threshold smaller nerves as well. According to *Melzack and Wall,* whether or not pain is perceived depends on the balance between large neuron input representing non-noxious sensation and small diameter neuron input involved in the perception of pain. If small neuron input predominates, the spinothalamic pathways fire and pain is perceived. If there is only large fiber input or if large fiber input predominates, the gate is closed and the pain is not perceived. Dominance of large fiber input can be obtained either by decreasing the noxious stimulus to reduce the small fiber contribution or by increasing the large fiber contribution. In its simplest terms, one can turn off or lessen pain by applying a non-painful stimulus.

When something hurts, we rub it to make it feel better. This universal practice relies on the theoretical gate. A non-noxious stimulus, rubbing, stimulates the large fibers, which in turn inhibit the transmission of a painful impulse. In a more scientific milieu, we may stimulate the skin electronically through electrodes taped to the skin at a voltage sufficient to cause a non-painful impulse, one which, by definition, stimulates the low threshold larger fibers but not the smaller high-threshold pain fibers. This process, called transcutaneous stimulation, will be discussed in detail later.

Suggested Reading

1   Liebeskind, J.C.; Paul, L.A.: Psychological and physiological mechanisms of pain. A. Rev. Physiol. *28:* 41–60 (1977).
2   Melzack, R.: The puzzle of pain (Penguin, Harmondsworth 1973).
3   Melzack, R.; Wall, P.: Pain mechanisms: a new theory. Science *150:* 971–979 (1965).

Chapter III

What Is Chronic Pain?

Much confusion in the doctor's office stems from the difference between *acute pain* and *chronic pain*. Acute pain results from the application of a noxious stimulus. A noxious or nociceptive stimulus is one which has the potential to produce or actually produces tissue damage. Examples of noxious stimuli include pin stick, pinch, heat, or electric shock of sufficient intensity. In clinical practice, noxious stimuli include mechanical damage such as occurs with fractures, lacerations, or other trauma. One of the hallmarks of inflammation is *dolor* or pain, which results from tissue stretching or distortion or chemical factors connected with the acute inflammatory process.

Acute pain is that which the neurophysiologists talk about when they apply a noxious stimulus in the laboratory to analyze the pain pathways. Consequently, most of what we know about the physiology of pain actually refers to acute pain.

When a patient comes into the office complaining of pain of recent onset, possibly of significant intensity, it can be assumed that there is some pathological process underlying the complaint and that the pain is 'acute'. Attention is directed to making the diagnosis, analyzing the process underlying the acute pain, and treating the etiologic condition. It is appropriate to assume that the pain is temporary and that it will go away when healing occurs. It is appropriate for the physician to direct his attention to the underlying disease process and to prescribe specific action to initiate the healing process.

All analgesic medications have been developed using acute pain as the experimental model. An animal is subjected to a painful stimulation and drugs administered to see if they can modify the response to that pain. However, virtually all analgesics lose their effectiveness as tolerance sets in when they are given over a period of time, and their effect on pain becomes much less. Consequently, it is appropriate to use analgesics in effective doses for the temporary management of acute pain, anticipating that the pain will subside before tolerance becomes well established. It is inappropriate, however, to assume that analgesics work for chronic pain, since they were never designed for that use.

Pain from malignancy has many of the characteristics of both chronic pain and acute pain, but requires management that is different from either one. The pain of malignancy represents continuous application of a noxious stimulus and continual renewal of acute pain. Therefore, management often includes such aspects of acute pain management as narcotic analgesics or treatment directed toward the underlying disease. Procedures to interrupt the pain pathways should be reserved for cancer pain. Yet, because of the attendant chronic distress and disability, as well as the accompanying stress and anxiety, many of the psychological components of chronic pain can be recognized. Since the management of pain secondary to malignancy differs significantly from the management of chronic pain, it should not be managed exclusively by the chronic pain program outlined herein. For these reasons, this book will address itself only to the management of chronic (not acute) pain, and not to the management of cancer pain.

Chronic pain, by definition, has persisted for a long time (we use 6 months as an arbitrary dividing line). There may or may not be an identifiable underlying disease process, or healing may have occurred, but the pain persists. Chronic pain serves no useful biologic function! The recognized pain pathways may not be involved in the perception of chronic pain, and interruption of those pathways ordinarily results in only transient relief of chronic pain. It is important to know this and to realize that cutting pain pathways and the usual analgesics are ineffective against chronic pain and may actually potentiate it.

Physicians who fail to appreciate the difference between an acute and chronic problem are often tempted to blame the patient if the cause for the continuation of pain is not found. All too often the physician's personal defenses may enter into play. He may conclude derisively that 'the pain is all in your head'. This attitude primarily massages the physician's ego, which is reeling from the insult of the patient's not behaving as expected by providing a readily diagnosable illness.

We must recognize sadly that medical education is almost exclusively geared to the concept of acute disease. The medical student is taught to 'take care of' the patient. The goal is to make a diagnosis of the underlying etiology, whether the symptom is pain or something else. Then, with brilliant diagnosis in hand, the physician launches an equally brilliant treatment program. If the patient responds and the disease is cured, the student learns that appropriate accolades are bestowed at the weekly conference. If the patient does not respond or the diagnosis turns out to be wrong, the blame is aired at the next morbidity and mortality conference. If no diagnosis becomes apparent and the patient continues to complain, he is very often pushed aside and forgotten while the physician sets out in more challenging and rewarding directions.

Lost in that shuffle is the acknowledgement that a sizable proportion of any physician's patients, regardless of his specialty, will be suffering from pain against which the usual medical school approach is ineffective. Many physicians, then, graduate from medical school to enter the world of medical practice poorly equipped for one of the most common challenges they will face, the practical management of chronic pain.

Again, it is important to recognize the difference between patients with acute pain and those with chronic pain, since correct management of these two groups is so different. In the chronic pain patient, no cure can be anticipated, or it would have been evident long before. Attention is directed not toward identifying and treating the underlying etiology (which should have been completed in the acute stage), but toward helping the patient cope with the resultant disability and side effects of medications. This takes the form of discontinuing addictive medications, treating depression and helping the patient change his attitude to move from regressed and dependent behavior toward initiative and independence. The change is effected through resocialization and remobilization. Specific modalities for the treatment of pain play a lesser role. They may be helpful as an adjunct part of the program, but certainly are rarely effective when used alone.

It is equally important for the physician to differentiate between pain and suffering. When pain occurs from a physical cause, such as an illness or injury, the immediate manifestation is the patient's awareness of the pain. If the pain is not promptly alleviated, there is an autonomic and emotional response as well, which may take the form of 'fight or flight', nausea, or gastrointestinal distress. Next comes the occurrence of suffering, as distinct from pain itself. This emotional distress, if long-standing, leads to depression and personality changes. Physicians must be aware that pain and suffering are separate events. Suffering may occur in the absence of pain (even though the patient may express it in somatic terms) or it may continue after the etiology and the associated physiologic pain have resolved.

The physician must not overlook the possibility that the patient's attention is so *squarely* directed to the chronic pain complaint that other physical problems are overlooked.

Chapter IV

Chronic Pain Patients –
What They Have in Common

Clinical medicine teaches us to expect that patients, even those with similar medical problems, will vary widely in their responses to illness and will often require very different kinds of management. Despite clinical experiences that reinforce this belief in 'how different people are' we have been startled to find that most chronic pain patients present in a remarkably similar way. Close observation and study of these similarities has enabled us to formulate a common and very basic principle in the evaluations of chronic pain patients – namely, they present as caricatures of acute patients, with the concerns, behaviors, and urgency for treatment that would be appropriate to the acutely ill. Again, confusion about the differences between chronic and acute illness by both patient and physician are a major source of frustration and disappointment in the treatment of this patient group.

Several common features of presentation emerged from clinical evaluations of over 300 patients with chronic pain.

– All, for instance, reported pain of months to years in duration.

– Most stated that the current pain was similar to their initial pain, which was usually associated with an acute medical problem or injury, but that it became worse following the many unsuccessful medical or surgical attempts at relief.

– They offered medical histories of treatment failures freely and in great detail, often with considerable relish.

– All had tried many medications and the majority were addicted to narcotics. They continued to take the various analgesics and tranquilizers despite their own testimonies that the medication offered neither significant nor long-lasting relief, but commented often that they took the medication 'to take the edge off' the pain.

– All presented their pain complaints as urgent or emergency problems. They described the pain as unbearable and incapacitating.
– They expressed, for the most part, willingness to undergo any treatment aimed at pain relief, believing that the pain had an as yet unidentified organic cause.
– Finally, many claimed they had no other problems and that everything would be fine if only the doctor would treat their pain. If pressed about the possibility of depression or personal, family or other concerns, they became defensive, allowing at most that if other problems existed they were consequences of the pain. The patient's daily life was organized around and defined by the pain; the pain explained all difficulties in living.

Physical examination and further questioning usually led evaluators to feel that the pain report was excessive for the physical findings and, therefore, that emotional factors contributed significantly to the perception of pain.

Presence of like histories in so many cases allowed us to draw a profile of the chronic pain patient in which the following features predominate:
– Presence of the kind of pain for which medical treatment cannot offer a reasonable expectation of cure.
– Lack of relief from medication and often depression, addiction or decreased ability to function normally as a result of overmedication.
– Disability in excess of that warranted by physical findings.
– Contribution of psychological and social factors to reinforcement and perpetuation of pain behavior.
– Overvaluation of the pain, i.e., the pain plays a central part in how the patients relate to themselves and others.
– Manipulation of others which, the histories reveal, has often succeeded in maneuvering physicians into attempting ill-advised medical or surgical procedures.
– Often the presence of medical illness unrelated to the pain and overlooked because of the patient's restricted focus on the pain complaint.

Pervading the history and presentation are a sense of urgency, assertions of distress and disability, and expectations that an illness will be named and a definitive treatment instituted. While these behaviors and expectations are understandable in patients with acute illness or injury, they are inappropriate when the problem is so obviously a chronic one. The incongruity between expectations and possible real outcome made it clear that the first step in constructive treatment would have to be weening

patients from the familiar treatment/cure expectations of acute care experiences. Patients themselves are not wholly responsible for their unrealistic
expectations. The acute treatment training and orientation of physicians
reinforces expectations for cure and, in the case of most chronic pain
patients, results in sanctioned chronic sick role occupancy.

*We believe that little in the way of pain management can be accom-
plished unless and until both patient and treating physician exchange the
goal of pain relief for that of rehabilitation.*

We contend that these patient profiles are an epiphenomenon of
assuming the acute sick role on a chronic basis. Temporary exemption from
responsibilities, with the regression and dependence it brings, can help the
patient accept the physician's recommendations. Long-term sick role occupancy, however (and it must be remembered that many of our patients
maintained sick role identity for years and years), distorts the function of
'normal' sick role occupancy. If we observe the behavior of the chronic pain
patient in light of the acute sick role expectations, the following distortions
become obvious.

A. Acutely Sick Patients Are Expected to Seek Medical Help

Pain patients' long histories of physician contacts and treatment failures are an outgrowth of the acute sick role obligation to seek medical help.
The implicit social expectation is that once medical help has been found,
the patient will be cured. When not cured, the chronic pain patient continues to seek medical help until the quest itself becomes a major preoccupation. Referrals to other physicians are often interpreted by the patient as
rejections. In the patient's view, furthermore, the referring physician is not
fulfilling his professional obligation.

One case illustrative of how seeking help can become more important
than the injury is that of a patient whose pain complaint began with a minor
procedure secondary to an ankle injury. The operation failed to produce
desired results, so a second was performed. Many more followed in rapid
succession, leading eventually to complete disability, drug addiction, and
marked regression. It was not until 15 years later that evaluation in our
clinic identified this individual as a chronic pain patient.

Patients' families very often participate in the search. The behavior of
patients and their families is completely in line with what is expected of the
acutely sick. Their disappointment at unrealized expectations is under-

standable within the frame of reference of the acutely ill. The reason for frustration (physicians' and patients') is misidentification of the problem as acute.

B. Patients Are Expected to Cooperate with Medical Management

Chronic pain patients usually volunteer that they will do whatever the doctor suggests to relieve their pain. This attitude reflects an implicit understanding that if patients 'do their job', i.e., be willing and cooperative, doctors will 'do their job' and cure the pain. For patients with chronic pain, cooperation often leads to excessive drug use and polypharmacy. In a controlled study of multiple surgery patients with chronic pain who were matched to psychiatric controls, we found that chronic pain patients were receiving four times the number of drugs (especially narcotics, analgesics and minor tranquilizers) as the control psychiatric patients. More significant was the pain patients' report that the medications were not particularly helpful. When asked why they continued ineffective drug treatment, they most commonly responded, 'My doctor told me to take it,' or 'I have to take something for the pain.' The taking of medication was more meaningful in conferring the status of 'sick' and 'need treatment' than as a palliative measure.

C. The Sick Are Expected to Want to Get Better

Despite evidence of regression, exaggerated disability and excessive drug use, chronic pain patients insist that they want to return to work and resume former responsibilities. Their expectations are most often expressed in such a manner as, 'As soon as the doctor fixes me up so I'm in the shape I was in before all this happened, I'll be able to take up where I left off.' Such statements deny the likelihood that other problems block return to work and reacceptance of responsibility. They deny also the possibility that the patient may not regain former health or use of the painful body part. The problem is still conceptualized by the patient as an acute one; one that need only be identified before the patient can be 'cured' and become his or her former self. The former self that is referred to may be as much as 10, 15 or even 20 years younger. Families share the patient's expectations of complete cure and share also in the search for the doctor who will effect it. Much of the frustration experienced by chronic caretakers comes from waiting for the eventual definitive treatment.

D. A Privilege of the Sick Is Exemption from Social Responsibilities

One declared sick by a physician is excused from responsibilities as spouse, parent, and wage earner and is cared for by others. It is not surprising that when exemption is prolonged, patients become less capable of resuming their former role duties. Inactivity and drug overuse lead to poor general health which, along with being cared for and relieved of responsibility, intensifies regression. Soon patients are unable to deal with the merest of everyday concerns.

The sick role offers the only socially sanctioned return to childhood. Sanctioned permission to avoid responsibility, be cared for, and enjoy the other rewards of being sick is referred to as *secondary gain,* and is an important variable in patient recovery or failure to recover. We feel, moreover, that many patients adapt very readily to the sick role because they are poorly equipped to handle adult responsibilities. In the sense that illness resolves a patient's conflict over inability to face adult responsibilities by sanctioning his exemption from them, it represents primary gain.

External incentives for non-recovery, such as compensation and disability payments or lawsuits, should be identified during patient evaluation. We have found patients particularly reluctant to cooperate with efforts at rehabilitation when insurance settlements or disability status will be adversely affected by their progress.

E. The Sick Are Entitled to Be Cared For

The right to be cared for and to become more child-like is a sanctioned privilege of the acute sick role. Its value as secondary gain and its contributions to both physical disablement and regression, however, make it counter-productive in chronic illness. When someone is diagnosed as sick, family members are conscripted as caretakers and share the former responsibilities of the patient. The evolution of caretakers from family members often follows the same course. At first the family is concerned and upset and willingly sacrifices normal routine and comfort to ease the patient's distress.

When sick role occupancy is protracted, family members either become frustrated and resent the continued need to sacrifice, or they develop a more comfortable adjustment in which the patient is treated like a child. Spouses of chronic pain patients often insist on being present during evaluation; many talk for the patient and appear in every way to be parents of small children. Patients can be so regressed as to be completely dependent upon spouse and children for the simplest of tasks. Working with the family to discourage regressed behavior and reinforce rehabilitative behavior is a major management intervention.

More must be said also of *psychological regression* – so great a factor in the disability of chronic pain patients. Regression is an expected response to acute illness. In medical patients, this return to a more child-like state is usually characterized by marked increase in egocentricity, reduced scope of interest, preoccupation with bodily perceptions, notable increase in dependency, and oftentimes a demanding and manipulative insistence upon attention. While these behaviors may actually enhance compliance and therefore recovery in acute illness, overly severe or prolonged regression seriously hampers the ability to cope with a chronic condition and to return to normal social functioning. It has been noted that the hospital environment fosters regression through enforced passivity, the uncertain meaning of medical diagnoses to patients, and the implied promise that if they are good their primitive needs will be met. The patient cannot resume the path to rehabilitation and independence while lying in bed having a nurse take care of him. Many of the undesirable characteristics of chronic pain patients can be understood when it is recognized that they are acting within the framework of these expectations. Repeated rehospitalization serves only to reinforce these characteristics.

The critically limited value of psychological assessment, particularly psychological testing, as a diagnostic tool is due, we think, to patient regression. For example, investigators have shown that *neurotic elevations on the MMPI scale do not discriminate accurately between pain of psychological origin and that of organic origin, nor do they predict response to surgical treatment.* Regressive symptomatology noted on psychological evaluation or translated into elevated neurotic MMPI profiles frequently leads to misdiagnoses of hypochondriasis, depression, or personality disorder. More likely, the symptoms and MMPI elevations simply bespeak the moderate to severe regression that is secondary to chronic sick role behavior.

The histories and presentation of chronic pain patients, then, are remarkably similar and are products of their preoccupying search for a definitive treatment for a non-curable pain. Their moderate to severe regression calls into question the value of the usual psychological tests as diagnostic or prognostic tools. When, through various strategies, patients are removed from the regressed position, specific diagnostic and prognostic judgments can be more reliably made. In our experience, the severity of the chronic pain problem (and therefore the difficulty in rehabilitation) ranges along a continuum and is based upon the intensity of the patient's need to be sick.

Suggested Reading

1   Ayd, F.J.: Treatment of the office neurotic. Clin. Symposia 9(5): 151–188 (1957).
2   DeVaul, R.A.; Hall, R.C.W.; Faillace, L.A.: Drug use by the polysurgical patient. Am. J. Psychiat. 135: 682–685 (1978).
3   Engel, G.L.: Psychogenic pain and the pain-prone patient. Am. J. Med. 26: 899–918 (1959).
4   Fordyce, W.E.: Pain viewed as learned behavior. Adv. Neurol. 4: 415–422 (1974).
5   Gunther, M.S.: Psychiatric consultation in rehabilitation hospital. A regression hypothesis. Compreh. Psychiat. 12: 572–585 (1971).
6   Kahana, R.J.; Bebring, G.L.: Personality types in medical management; in Zinberg, Psychiatry and medical practice in a general hospital, pp. 108–123 (International University Press, New York 1964).
7   Menninger, K.A.: Polysurgery and polysurgical addiction. Polyanaly. Quart. 3: 173–199 (1934).
8   Owen, W.H.P.: Pills for personal problems. Br. med. J. 27: 749–751 (1975).
9   Parsons, T.: The social system, pp. 428–479 (Free Press, New York 1951).
10 Peterson, B.H.: Psychological reactions to acute physical illness in adults. Med. J. Aust. i: 311–316 (1974).
11 Sargent, D.A.: Confinement and ego regression: some consequences of enforced passivity. Int. J. Psych. Med. 5: 143–151 (1974).
12 Sternbach, R.A.: Pain and depression; in Kiev, Somatic manifestations of depressive disorders (Excerpta Medica, New York 1974).
13 Wahl, C.W.; Golden, J.S.: The psychodynamics of the polysurgical patient. Report of sixteen patients. Psychosomatics 7: 65–72 (1966).
14 Weintraub, M.I.: Hysteria. A clinical guide to diagnosis. Clin. Symposia 29(6): 2–31 (1977).

Chapter V

Types of Chronic Pain Patients

Generally, patients with chronic pain can be divided into four categories (table I).

A. The Need-to-Suffer Patient. Some people have a psychological need to suffer. They present to the physician with a complaint of chronic pain, but it becomes apparent through a thorough history-taking that they have bounced from one situation to another where they have placed themselves into the posture of suffering. It is important to recognize these patients, since they are so often treated inappropriately or with unjustified invasive techniques which eventually fail or make them fulfill an unconscious goal to suffer more.

B. The Overwhelmed Patient. By far the largest percentage of patients that we see in the Chronic Pain Clinic are those who have occupied the sick role as a response to overwhelming problems. Although physical problems may have precipitated their decompensation, once they have established

Table I. General types of pain patients in chronic sick role occupancy

	A The need-to-suffer patient	B The overwhelmed patient	C The psychogenic patient	D The assigned patient	
Greatest difficulty with rehabilitation	←			→	Least difficulty with rehabilitation
	lifelong personality disorder (20)[1]	premorbid function marginal (70)[1]	premorbid function varies (5)[1]	premorbid function good (5)[1]	

[1] Estimated number of patients per 100 seen in pain clinic.

the pattern of sick role behavior, emotional problems become involved, so that a combination of physical and psychological factors is responsible for the resulting distress.

C. The Psychogenic Patient. A very small percentage of chronic pain patients are those who have purely psychogenic pain. They may have a premorbid personality problem, or may be responding to an emotionally troubling event which may or may not be associated with the trauma producing an injury.

D. The Assigned Patient. A few patients get into the chronic pain-disability rut because their physicians have inadvisably assigned them to that role. These patients may require only redefinition of their roles to overcome their problems and this can be done quite readily by the knowledgeable family doctor.

A. The Need-to-Suffer Patient

A number of patients can be thought of as having a personality that indicates a need to suffer. While they represent only a minority of chronic pain patients, members of this group are responsible for most of the frustration and disappointment associated with chronic pain management. They have been variously described in the psychiatric literature as pain-prone personalities, masochistic personalities, and 'crocks'. Common to these designations is recognition of a life-long pervasive personality style that is characterized by pain and suffering and resists the lessons of experience.

Pain is a psychological necessity to members of this group. Unlike the groups of chronic pain patients – those on whom sick role occupancy is imposed, those for whom it meets a current understandable need, and those with psychogenic pain – this group uses sickness to fill a life-long need to suffer. Early identification of such patients and management strategies designed to reduce the overtreatment, frustration, and disappointment that result from acute treatment attempts are important to emphasize. A typical case history and discussion of a 'need-to-suffer' patient illustrates how clinical evidence is accumulated to suggest a diagnosis:

Mrs. K., a 40-year-old white married mother of two, was admitted to the general surgery unit of a university teaching hospital for evaluation of abdominal pain. At that time, she was taking large doses of meperidine and several tranquilizers. She had a history of abdominal operations. Initial medical evaluation, including laboratory and X-ray screening, was negative with the exception of her pain report upon palpation of the abdomen in general. The pain became more severe despite increased doses of narcotics and tranquilizers, while objective tests continued to yield negative results. The patient denied having any difficulties other than the pain for which she was seeking treatment.

The clinical picture, thus far, is similar to that of many chronic pain patients – a focusing on the pain complaint, denial of other personal problems, and insistence that everything would be all right if the doctor would simply cure the pain. Often the urgency in presentation leads to abbreviated history-taking and immediate attempts at palliative pain relief.

When asked further about the pain, Mrs. K. was not only willing to discuss it, but was comfortable and engaging during her report of medical treatments and surgeries aimed at pain relief. Interviews with family members brought to light information which suggested that Mrs. K. faced many personal, family, and financial problems.

Upon this evidence, the pain complaint might be suspected as having psychological origin or, at least, components. The presentation is compatible with that of pain secondary to depression, pain as a symptom of conversion neurosis or pain used to gain sick-role status and release from the unwanted responsibilities of healthy adulthood. Differential diagnosis from among these and other possibilities is based on further details of the medical history and upon a full social history of the patient's early life.

Mrs. K. revealed that she had undergone 20 operations and countless medical treatments for the same pain. Moreover, the circumstances surrounding each of the surgeries were strikingly similar. Each time, the patient had been told by a surgeon that the pain did not warrant surgery, and each time she had been able to find another surgeon who, claiming significant evidence of pathology, would operate for the pain. The pain always returned a few days after surgery, leading Mrs. K. to angry separation from each of the physicians. All in all, the pain had persisted for 20 years.

The pain onset, then, is not tied to current or circumstantial causes. The social history confirms the impression that a personality style with a need to suffer underlies the enduring pain symptom.

Mrs. K. was the youngest of 9 children. Her parents were overwhelmed by the burden of supporting and caring for the large family. She recalled having to work hard as a child and remembered receiving affection only when ill or after beatings which she would provoke in order to elicit her parents' guilty attention. She related a life-long history of suffering. In her own words, 'My life reads like a bad novel'. She was physically abused by her father and left home at an early age to marry an older alcoholic. The first of her abdominal operations occurred during her late adolescence. She did not report being bothered by the pain during times of external problems and stress but volunteered that pain or illness returned 'just when everything was going well'. Repeated therapeutic failures and disillusionment with successive physicians neither deterred her from seeking further treatment nor dimmed her hope that another physician would be able to cure her.

For all their seeming uniqueness, the details of Mrs. K.'s history are common identifying features in most chronic pain secondary to a need to suffer.

– The style of medical presentation, that is, the patient's need to recount the disappointments of previous medical encounters, is itself the first clue. Physicians are often put off from the patient's recital by the press of office activities, the apparent urgency of the pain complaint, or their own need to structure the interview so as to get what they feel is more relevant information. Patients' desires to present their sagas of disappointment and suffering, along with the content of these sagas, are, in truth, very relevant. Listening carefully, one is impressed with the patients' common needs to present themselves as long-suffering and abused. They are nevertheless willing to put themselves in the care of yet another physician and have exaggerated hopes of success. Physicians might initially feel, along with sympathy for the patient's excessive misfortune, professional discomfort that medicine has failed to offer any significant pain relief. When reflected upon, however, the history and presentation yield several facts important to diagnosis. Most obvious is that the patient's pain is not acute but is of long standing and has a complicated supporting medical history. There is also some obvious disparity between the patient's apparent current general health and physical well-being on the one hand, and the somewhat exaggerated presentation of intractable pain, previous misfortunes, and suffering on the other. The patient is oftentimes well-dressed, engaging, and more than willing to discuss the many trials in a stoic, almost social, fashion. The attentive physician will turn next to the social and medical histories to confirm characteristics of a personality with a need to suffer.

– The patient frequently is from a large family where deprivation, hard work and physical abuse were routine. Not uncommonly, the father was an alcoholic and patients admit receiving verbal or physical abuse in early childhood. The mother very often had many illnesses and pain complaints. Patients may recall their own illnesses as times of respite from hard work and as rare occasions of affection from parents. There is usually evidence that in early and later important relationships the patient provoked abuse in order to receive affection born of guilt.

The lives of these patients, chaotic overall, appear at first to be series of tragedies and unrealized fantasies. Tragic losses and serial marriages to abusing spouses are commonplace. Under further analysis, many of the tragic situations are shown to be events over which the patient could have exercised some control and did not. Likewise, the many instances of 'ill fortune' occurred because patients repeatedly placed themselves in situations which had turned out badly for them in the past and would eventually do so again.

–   Careful consideration of the onset of pain and the pattern of its recurrence and exacerbation is equally rewarding diagnostically. Pain symptoms frequently begin in childhood or adolescence, with patterns of painful illness and medical intervention developing over the years. In one observed pattern, patients develop illnesses and undergo surgeries similar to those of a parent, particularly the mother. One such patient experienced the same operations (including hysterectomy, gallbladder removal and successive surgeries for abdominal adhesions) at the same time in her life as her mother had experienced them. As we saw in the case of Mrs. K., events surrounding the successive medical and surgery interventions can also become patterned.

A hallmark of this group is the pattern of pain recurrence and exacerbation. Most people, including other types of chronic pain patients, recognize that they are more likely to become ill when they are having personal problems or are under stress. In contrast, patients with a need to suffer seem to function best when life circumstances are most stressful. They seldom recall having pain symptoms during their many bouts with bad luck and external crises. On the other hand, they often report having to seek medical attention for illness or pain when other aspects of their lives were most satisfactorily under control. This deserves emphasis because this is the only patient group in which the phenomenon is noted.

–   Evidence of a need to suffer can be found in the details of the doctor-patient relationship. The patient has a need to relate a history in which he or she appears long-suffering, and the similarity of the patient's interaction with successive physicians is often a pattern. The pattern is usually one in which the physician attempts to reassure the patient and offer symptomatic relief. The reassurance is rejected and the attempts at relief of symptoms fail. It is particularly helpful diagnostically to note that such patients rarely, if ever, gain relief from narcotics. The disappointed patient eventually seeks another physician, although not, perhaps, until another surgery has been performed and has failed to cure the pain. When patients report no pain relief or worse pain after reasonable therapeutic attempts and when, at the same time, objective support for a diagnosis of organic etiology fails to appear, physicians should investigate the possibility that their patients are members of the 'need-to-suffer' group. Should the underlying personality style go unrecognized, the spiral of treatment/increased pain widens to include ever more extreme treatments and surgeries.

Physicians must understand the patient's need to suffer in order to design rational and constructive management interventions. The personality style of this patient group is based upon a pervasive and exaggerated guilt. As children they were poorly treated and often materially and emotionally deprived. They accepted guilt as an explanation for the treatment and the grim world they viewed. This led to a masochistic character, that is, one which must suffer in order to feel deserving of affection. The long-suffering and self-sacrificing behavior pattern seen in these people represents atonement for guilt. Much of their behavior in relationships to important others, including the physician, can be understood as an expression of the belief that, 'I must suffer in order to have a relationship', or 'You must care for me because I suffer so terribly'.

This belief lies behind not only their need to present themselves as long-suffering, but also their deprecating behavior and their use of pain as a way to atone for guilt. When external crises offer a mechanism for suffering and atonement, pain symptoms often subside.

Physicians, whose training and professional goals revolve around relieving pain, find it difficult both to understand and to deal with patients whose pain is necessary to their way of functioning. Not only is the pain necessary, but it is viewed by these patients as the major justification for their desired relationship with the physician. The clinical clues just outlined make recognition of the personality that indicates a need to suffer relatively easy, and recognition should interrupt the pattern of escalating treatments. Effective management, in fact, will require the physician to give up the idea of cure or even significant pain relief. A realistic and constructive approach with this group is to represent their reacceptance of social responsibility (including work and family responsibilities) as yet another burden, that is, another opportunity to suffer.

Like all chronic pain patients, members of this group must first be confronted with the nature of their chronic pain. They should also be told that there is, unfortunately, no definitive treatment for such pain and that, as they can testify, pain medications are ineffective. Mobilization and resumption of their social role obligations should then be presented as tasks that must be attempted for the benefit of those who depend upon them. If medication is indicated for clinically significant depression, for example, it should be offered not as a pain reliever or cure, but as something that might be of help to them in their effort to carry on. Physicians should express willingness to continue to see the patient at regular intervals, independent of changes in the patient's pain report. Regular appointments, whether the patient is feeling well or ill, should be planned with the hope of demonstrating that suffering is not a prerequisite for receiving the physician's attention.

Finally, the primary concern with this group, as with other chronic pain patients, is to protect them from unnecessary medical and surgical procedures and iatrogenic drug dependence. These undesirable consequences are so often products of the clash between antithetical needs – the physician's, to relieve suffering, and the patient's, to suffer.

B. The Overwhelmed Patient

Chronic pain may be a response to overwhelming problems. Even prior to their pain these patients had found it stressful to cope with adult life. Frequently, they have had a history of irresponsible behavior. There is a large incidence of job dissatisfaction – any job. They may have used other means to escape from responsibility in the past, and there is a high incidence of alcohol abuse. They go through life feeling put upon and stressed and would like nothing better than to escape.

Then one day, escape comes. It may be in the form of an injury or illness which causes temporary confinement, which the patient may find quite agreeable. It may be in the form of an accident at work, which may prove to be a bonanza. Not only can the patient escape the responsibility of working and making adult decisions, but can do so without giving up the fruits of work, with a guaranteed disability income as long as the pain continues. The system we have for compensating the disabled could not have been designed more efficiently to promote disability. It is based on the fallacy that the greatest motivation people have is to work. Actually, the greatest motivation that most people have is to be paid, and, if they can accomplish that without working, so much the better.

The structure of the disability system is set up along classical operant conditioning lines. A specified behavior (having pain) is rewarded (disability payments). As long as pain behavior continues, it is reinforced with the appropriate reward. If the response disappears (getting better) the reward is withdrawn (denial of disability payments).

The result is that the individual at that time must change his status from being disabled to returning to the work force. Ordinarily, this is a hoped for and anticipated transition. What happens, however, when the patient is unable to accept adult responsibility? Such patients have only one other logical option – to remain disabled (in pain).

Perhaps one of the most difficult situations with which to deal concerns the patient who has the need to escape from adult responsibility and has a spouse who encourages his regressed behavior. The patient feels the need to behave as a child and to develop a dependency type of relationship, and the spouse has the need to have the patient dependent on him or her, either becuase the spouse feels threatened by a more mature type of relationship (since the spouse may feel the threat of abandonment if the patient is independent), or to satisfy parenteral instincts. When two people have such an abnormal means for fulfilling their emotional needs, it is often much more than coincidence which brings them together in marriage.

The classical situation concerns a marriage that may not have been doing well. The children may be grown, leaving the wife feeling depressed and useless. The husband may be restless in the marriage, may be cheating, or may not be mature enough to sustain a satisfactory marital relationship. In addition, he may have difficulties fulfilling the responsibilities of being the head of the household, including financial survival and decision-making. The relationship may be floundering until the husband is injured, preferably at work.

There is a sudden shift in the relationship to a level which both partners find much more satisfactory. The husband must no longer fend for himself in the real world. The responsibility of making a living may be taken care of automatically through disability payments. The husband is suddenly less threatened by the marriage, since much of the burden of responsibility has been lifted. As he becomes more disabled, he regresses to a more infantile and dependent state, which he finds more comfortable.

While the husband regresses, the wife assumes a more commanding role. She no longer fears her husband's departure, and can be more positive and aggressive toward him which he, in his newly regressed state, can accept. The wife assumes the role of a mother. She feels fulfilled and he feels comfortable, having escaped from adult responsibility.

What if he were suddenly to lose his pain? Would he have to return to the adult responsibilities with which he could not cope? Would the marriage revert to the previously unacceptable relationship? Would the wife find herself once again threatened and unfulfilled? Would their newly found contentment be marred by the recurrence of prior conflicts? You don't have to tune in tomorrow to know what the answers will be. The new relationship, although not the social norm, is more psychologically satisfactory for both spouses. However, it must be recognized that an important ingredient in this new relationship is chronic pain, and the relationship cannot exist without it. While the physician's goal may be to remove the pain, both the patient and his wife recognize (but may not vocalize) that the satisfactory relationship depends on the presence of chronic pain, and both will do everything to perpetuate the pain. Indeed, the husband may find the physical pain much less disagreeable than the prior emotional pain!

C. The Psychogenic Patient

The parts played by psychological and social factors in the perception and maintenance of pain have been discussed. In addition to those factors already mentioned, stress is a common contributor to pain complaints, accompanied, as it frequently is, by a focusing on bodily concerns and by tension symptoms such as headache, backache, and exaggerated perception of existing organic symptoms. There exist, apart from pain symptoms which are maintained or magnified by psychological, social, and stress factors, pain symptoms of pure psychological origin. Such pain is referred to as *psychogenic pain.* Psychogenic pain is a real perception with many of the same physiological concomitants of organic pain. Such soft neurological findings as paresthesias and functional motor weakness (Walter's psychogenic regional pain) are not unusual, and neither placebo trial nor psychological testing is reliable in differentiating this pain from that of organic origin. The similarities between organic and psychogenic pain place patients with the latter at risk for unnecessary and inappropriate medical procedures, including investigative tests, surgeries, and iatrogenic drug dependence.

The most reliable tools for identifying patients with psychogenic pain are an extensive medical history and close observation of the patient's clinical presentation. Based upon these two sources of information, diagnosis of the pain as one of five, relatively well-defined, types of psychogenic pain can usually be made. The subgroups of psychogenic pain are (1) pain as a symptom of depression, (2) pain as a delusional symptom of psychosis, (3) pain as a symptom of anxiety, (4) pain as a conversion of hysterical neurosis, and (5) pain as a symptom of unresolved grief. The following discussion of the five subgroups of psychogenic pain includes an explanation of the origin of pain in each description of a typical clinical presentation with emphasis on the identifying characteristics and, finally, suggestions for management.

1. Pain as a Symptom of Depression

Depression, like stress, is ordinarily accompanied by heightened self-concern and awareness of the body. Pain complaints, therefore, are common in clinical depression. Depressive patients may be preoccupied with and complain exclusively of the pain. Only direct questioning about specific alterations in the patient's behavior exposes the underlying problem. Patients and their families should be asked whether the patient has been feeling 'down' or 'blue', they have become easily fatigued, been unable to concentrate, lost interest and satisfaction in work, become unable to function efficiently, withdrawn from family and friends, had unprovoked crying spells, experienced sleep disturbance (especially early morning awakening), been constipated, lost weight or appetite, lost interest in sex, or thought about suicide. It is also important to inquire about past depressions (particularly any which required hospitalization), history of alcoholism or accident-proneness, and previous episodes of hyperactivity or manic behavior. Family history of depression, alcoholism or sociopathy should be noted.

Mild to severe depression frequently accompanies chronic organic pain. When a pain complaint is coupled with symptoms of depression, therefore, the diagnostic task is to distinguish between psychogenic pain of depressive origin and depression secondary to chronic pain. Making the distinction is critical to successful management and is done by establishing the relative chronology of pain onset and onset of depression. This is sometimes a difficult task and requires very careful history-taking and attention to all events in the patient's life at or near the time the complaint originated. If considerable doubt remains after thorough questioning of patients and their families and the pain report has no apparent organic etiology, a trial of antidepressants and further psychiatric evaluation is recommended.

Mr. Y., a 52-year-old white married accountant, father of three, was admitted to the surgery service with a chief complaint of severe continuous left upper quadrant abdominal pain of 3 weeks' duration. Medical evaluation, including complete laboratory and X-ray survey, was negative. During the initial history-taking the patient presented only his pain symptom. Further history, obtained from the patient and his family upon direct questioning, however, contained evidence of a 3-month long increasing depression: early morning awakening, loss of appetite, a 20-pound weight loss, social withdrawal, unprovoked crying spells, and occasional suicidal ideation. The patient responded to tricyclic antidepressant treatment with complete pain relief.

This clinical picture characterizes pain of depressive origin, one of the more common types of psychogenic pain. The patient focused on the 'medical' complaint. The underlying depression was exposed through careful history-taking and close questioning of the patient and his family. Disappearance of pain following treatment for depression is also typical. In most cases, clinical depression responds to a 3-week trial treatment with tricyclic antidepressants administered in the 100- to 200-mg/day range. Response indicates that the treatment should be continued for about 2 months. It makes little difference which tricyclic antidepressant is used so long as adequate doses are taken over a long enough period of time. Physician familiarity with the drug and observation of the patient are important in light of possible anticholinergic side-effects that can aggrevate such clinical conditions as acute angle glaucoma and prostatism, and may induce cardiac arrhythmias.

Interestingly, patients with chronic pain without overt manifestations of depression may also respond to tricyclic antidepressants, suggesting a direct effect of the drugs on mechanisms of chronic pain perception.

Psychiatric consultation is advised if the patient fails to respond to tricyclic antidepressants or if the physician is unfamiliar with the treatment of clinical depression. Electroconvulsive therapy has been used effectively in some depressions refractory to antidepressant treatment.

2. Pain as a Delusional Symptom of Psychosis

A delusion is a fixed belief resistant to any real, natural or medical evidence that contradicts it. Delusional pain is the perception of a pain usually believed by the patient to be the result of some mechanical and unnatural cause. It can occur in any illness where perception of reality is impaired, including psychiatric disorders such as schizophrenia, hysterical psychosis, manic depressive psychosis, and clinical depression, and in organic brain syndromes such as toxic and withdrawal delirium. Delusional patients may describe bizarre, medically improbable or impossible causes for their pains, often giving them symbolic presentation or meaning. That is to say, the body part affected or the believed cause often has special meaning in the patient's emotional life.

Diagnosis of delusional pain in less disturbed, less outrightly psychotic patients is not always easily made in the structured medical interview. Intensive history-taking and oblique questioning of these patients will usually reveal their chaotic mental state and loss of contact with reality. When routine physical examination rules out medical cause for the pain complaint and preliminary or extensive interviewing suggests psychogenic pain of delusional origin, the patient should be referred to a psychiatrist. Frequently, appropriate antipsychotic treatment (in cases of psychosis) or treatment of the underlying condition (e.g., toxic delirium) leads to disppearance of the delusional pain and other symptoms of psychosis.

Mr. L. is a 21-year-old white single machinist, admitted to the psychiatric service with a complaint of persistent burning pain in his right shoulder caused by 'cosmic rays being broadcast by the local radio station'. The patient's presentation and history suggested the diagnosis of schizophrenic psychosis. He had received an electrical burn on his right shoulder at the age of six while working in his father's workshop. Treatment with antipsychotic doses of phenothiazines effected resolution of the patient's acute psychosis and pain.

Mrs. A. is a 48-year-old white married mother of three, admitted for a routine D and C. 3 days after her admission, she developed symptoms of alcohol withdrawal and acute delirium which went undiagnosed. Meanwhile she began to complain of severe thoracic pain which she described as 'ants eating my lungs'. When no organic etiology was demonstrated for the bizzare pain complaint, psychiatric consultation was ordered. During the psychiatric interview her disorientation and delirious state became evident. A withdrawal regimen and treatment with minor tranquilizers brought return of normal mental status and the subsequent disappearance of the pain complaint.

These cases of psychogenic pain of delusional origin responded to treatment of the pre-existing disorder, in the former case, psychosis, and in the latter, acute delirium.

3. Pain as a Symptom of Anxiety

Acute anxiety can, like depression and stress, cause heightened body awareness. In the case of acute anxiety, however, this is frequently attended by a nonspecific fearfulness which, in turn, brings on exaggerated concern over symptoms of medical distress. One particularly common medical by-product of acute anxiety is chest pain secondary to hyperventilation. When anxiety reaches panic proportions, patients may subconsciously begin to hyperventilate. Hyperventilation sets off a series of reactions – deficiency of carbon dioxide and a change in the acid/base balance in the blood, resulting changes in the ratio of bound to unbound calcium, and, finally, neuromuscular disturbances. Among the most commonly seen neuromuscular symptoms are a feeling of impending doom, paresthesias (particularly tingling around the mouth, hands and feet), an inability to catch one's breath and, oftentimes, constricting substernal chest pain.

Presence or absence of pre-existing acute anxiety is the major clue to differentiating between angina pain and pain brought on by anxiety. Both diagnoses are made on the basis of patient history and presentation. Two considerations predominate in making a differential diagnosis. (1) Can it be demonstrated that anxiety symptoms, the 'inability to catch a breath' or hyperventilation, preceded the onset of chest pain? If so, pain secondary to anxiety and hyperventilation is the likely diagnosis. If these symptoms did not precede the pain, angina might be more readily suspected. (2) Does the patient respond to the pain perception by becoming very still or does he respond by moving about, usually to open a window or 'get some fresh air'? The former behavior suggests angina; the latter, pain brought on by reaction to acute anxiety. As with the pain/depression relationship, anxiety can be secondary to angina just as chest pain can be secondary to anxiety, and, as with the former relationship, the sequence of events is the signal clue.

Mr. L. is a 53-year-old white married mechanic, father of three, who presented to the chronic pain service with a history of severe intermittent substernal chest pain of approximately 6 months' duration. He had been hospitalized on three occasions for cardiac evaluation, once in a cardiac intensive care unit for possible myocardial infarction. Laboratory evidence and EKG monitoring were negative. A careful review of Mr. L.'s history revealed that his pain had begun shortly after he was promoted from mechanic to garage manager. Although he felt very uncomfortable dealing with customer complaints, his employer refused to allow him to return to his former position. Finally the patient began to have episodes in wich he felt shortness of breath, tingling and cramping in his fingers and toes and substernal pain. The last sensation caused him particular concern because his father had recently died of a heart attack. The patient consulted a physician immediately. By the time he came to the pain clinic, the episodes had become more frequent, although tests for cardiac disease were still negative. After thorough history-taking, the diagnosis of anxiety with hyperventilation was made.

As in this case, which is typical of the fairly common clinical phenomenon, a situation can usually be identified which precipitates the onset of anxiety. Where anxiety can be established as the primary cause of pain, a two-step approach to management is indicated. The patient should first be made to understand the physiological chain of events responsible for the pain. After explaining the response mechanism, the physician might ask the patient to overbreathe there in the office to demonstrate that hyperventilation does, in fact, bring on the symptoms. Secondly, the patient is told how to manage the hyperventilation episode itself. Hyperventilation, when triggered by anxiety and the sense of fearfulness described above, is the body's preparation for increased activity that defense or survival may demand. For this reason, engaging in real activity, a brisk walk, for instance, can help regulate the breathing. The most satisfactory intervention is forestalling the anxiety reaction before hyperventilation begins. This can be done if patients relax completely or hold their breath momentarily. Often assurance that hyperventilation causes the pain enables patients to control overbreathing by this latter method.

4. Pain as a Symptom of Hysterical Neurosis

In hysterical neuroses, pain symptoms represent attempts to resolve personal conflict that the patient cannot deal with in a healthy way. Such symptoms are called conversion symptoms because early psychoanalytic investigators believed that repressed psychic energy, unexpressed as affect, was converted to somatic expression. Although belief in two separate kinds of energy has lost support, conversion symptoms are still recognized as symbolic physical expressions of, and solutions to, neurotic conflict.

Because of this, the symptoms are goal-oriented. A particular pain, for example, makes it impossible for the patient to carry out a certain role that would be odious or unacceptable. Other typical features in the presentation of conversion pain include (1) pain description that relates to an underlying personal conflict, (2) indifference to the pain despite its continued presence, (3) sudden onset of pain in an emotionally charged situation, (4) pain description that defies neuroanatomical boundaries, and (5) evidence of benefits gained by virtue of the pain disability, i.e., gratification of dependency needs or sanctioned release from responsibilities the patient would find impossible or repugnant in health.

Any personal or interpersonal conflict can become occasion for the production of conversion symptoms (of which pain is becoming the most common) provided the patient can neither consciously face the dilemma nor accept the responsibilities which healthy resolution of the conflict would impose. Typical conflictual settings include those of marital discord and other family and sex-related problems, job difficulties, and nonrecovery from traumatic injury, particularly where there are disability or compensation issues.

Miss D., a 14-year-old white high school student, was admitted to the surgery service for investigation of her complaint of crampy lower abdominal pain. History revealed that the patient's pain had begun suddenly in a setting of conflict with her mother. Miss D. wanted to have a baby and was unable to deal with her sexual feelings and the moral conflicts involved. The abdominal pain, which she described as like that of being in labor, at once symbolized her wishes and made it impossible for her to carry them out. The patient appeared relatively unconcerned about the pain and was noted to be seductive and manipulative. Physical examination and laboratory and X-ray evaluations were negative. This, coupled with details of the history and presentation, led to a diagnosis of conversion pain. Despite the diagnosis and the patient's relative indifference to the pain, the insistence on her part, and on her mother's, that something was seriously wrong led to an unnecessary laparotomy with negative findings.

When conversion pain is suspected, psychiatric evaluation, hypnosis or amytal interview may help confirm the diagnosis. Placebo medication is often misused in differential diagnosis of conversion pain because of lack of understanding of the placebo effect. This effect, which is powerful, derives from the complex sets of expectations that both patient and physician bring to the doctor/patient interaction. A significant part of all medical interventions, the placebo effect may be more useful in relieving peripheral organic pain (pain the patient wishes to be rid of) than in relieving conversion pain (pain the patient needs). For this reason, *placebo trial is not useful in differentiating physiological pain from conversion pain.* In addition, fooling the patient jeopardizes the trust essential to all constructive medical intervention.

Successful management of patients with conversion pain can be difficult. First, the physician should reassure the patient that there is no evidence of serious medical illness or pathology, and should express confidence that the symptom will be short-lived. It goes without saying that a physical examination and history and appropriate tests if necessary should be sufficiently thorough to convince both doctor and patient that organic pathology is unlikely. A minor analgesic may be prescribed with reassurance that it will probably relieve the pain. This approach is particularly effective with acute symptoms of recent, sudden onset. Patients who fail to respond to reassurance and suggestion should be confronted with the lack of evidence of organic illness. The patient can be told that there is no doubt about the validity of the pain and suffering, but that the pain is not the result of present tissue damage or disease and return to activity is advised. Explaining that the pain is largely a manifestation of stress usually elicits responses of perplexity, anger and disappointment, after which the patient may be willing to discuss personal problems and may agree to counseling or social intervention. It is critical to satisfactory management of patients with conversion pain that the physician demonstrate genuine concern and willingness to follow the patient, even when referrals are made to other sources of help.

5. Pain as a Symptom of Unresolved Grief

The grief and mourning that follow the death of a close relative or friend are part of a normal, necessary process. When grieving progresses properly, the bereaved pass through different stages, experiencing many emotions until finally their grief is resolved and they have the desire and ability to get on with their lives. Those who are unable to grieve at all, or to work through the entire grieving process, are at increased risk for mental illness.

Not uncommonly, in the early stage of grief, the bereaved identify temporarily with the deceased and their illnesses. If the bereaved cannot move beyond this stage, identification may continue and become pathological. In this form of unresolved grief, patients seek medical help for symptoms which they describe in the exact terms used to describe the illness of the deceased. Such patients are usually easily identified. Questioning about family deaths is a part of history-taking. When the death of a close relative is revealed, the patient should be asked, 'What was your response to the death? Did you attend the funeral? Do you still feel a need to cry for the deceased? Do you feel you have gotten over your grief for the individual?' Unresolved grief should be suspected when the patient spontaneously breaks into tears and admits that discussion of the loss is too painful, or, even more characteristically, when the patient 'dry tears', expressing both a need and an inability to cry.

Mrs. L. is a 24-year-old white married mother of two, admitted to the medical service with intermittent substernal chest pain of 2 months' duration. The diagnosis of angina was made on the basis of history. Further history revealed that the patient's mother had died quite suddenly of a heart attack approximately 2 weeks before the patient's symptoms began. Mrs. L. had been unable to attend the funeral, cry, or accept the fact that her mother was dead. Her description of her pain was identical to her description of her mother's. With encouragement Mrs. L. was able to begin grieving, and the chest pain disappeared.

The presentation of the pain complaint, like that of the deceased, is the hallmark of pain of unresolved grief, although the symptoms may take other forms as well. Further confirmation can be sought in a history-taking which includes the kinds of questions asked above. When unresolved grief is recognized to be the origin of a psychogenic pain complaint, initiation (or reinitiation) of grieving is the immediate management goal. It is best accomplished through regular counseling sessions with a family physician, minister or priest, or a social worker. During the sessions, the patient is made to talk about the deceased and encouraged to express all the intense, varied and confusing emotions associated with grief. Once mobilized, the grieving process will usually proceed as long as supportive listening and encouragement continue. Because grieving is painful and has been avoided by patients with grief-related facsimile illness, it is expected that they will feel worse before they feel better.

D. The Assigned Patient

There is a small group of patients who become chronic pain patients because they believe that is what is expected of them. Most often, they have been the victims of an accident, usually industrial.

Mr. A was struck on the shoulder by a falling crate while he was working as a warehouse manager. He went to his doctor who noted considerable bruising of the area, prescribed an oral narcotic-based analgesic, and ordered an X-ray, which was negative. 2 weeks later, Mr. A. returned to the doctor, at which time he still had limitation of motion and muscle spasm at the base of the neck. His doctor wrote a letter to Mr. A.'s employer, indicating that he anticipated that he would be disabled for an additional 6 weeks, and renewed his narcotic prescription. During that time, Mr. A. underwent physical therapy, but continued to have a moderate amount of pain.

6 weeks later, Mr. A. returned to his physician who asked about his condition, 'My shoulder still hurts and it still feels stiff', was Mr. A.'s reply. However, he failed to mention that the pain was really much better and that he was able to get by with minimal restriction of his activities. The response from the physician with no further questions or examination, was a renewal of the narcotic and another letter declaring Mr. A. disabled for an additional 2 months. Although Mr. A. felt that he might be able to return to work, he felt that the doctor knew better and, since his income continued, 'why not'?

This scene was repeated at 6-week intervals for almost a year, until the Worker's Compensation insurance carrier requested a second opinion. The second physician examined Mr. A. in much more detail and inquired about the severity of his pain. When he was told that the pain was not severe enough to interfere with Mr. A.'s activities, he suggested that Mr. A. return to work and discontinued his pain medication. Although Mr. A. had an uncomfortable week following the cessation of his narcotics, he was able to return to work successfully, and readily accepted the reassignment of his status.

Mr. A had been assigned to the role of a chronic pain patient by his initial physician who never made the transition from thinking of Mr. A. as an acute pain patient. He assigned him to the role as a patient because he still had symptoms, by that time on the basis of recurrent withdrawal. Mr. A., as a conscientious patient, never questioned his doctor, but accepted the role. He just as readily accepted the role that he was assigned by the second physician, which was much more appropriate to his actual physical condition.

Although it seems inconceivable that such patients may go for months assigned inappropriately to the role of a chronic pain patient, we have seen a number of these patients, even eventually referred to the Pain Clinic. Such patients most often accept their reassignment and return to normal activity with only a moderate amount of persuasion.

Although specific cause of pain differs, the presentation and management of patients with all five types of psychogenic pain is similar enough to allow a few general summary remarks. Most patients with psychogenic pain are not satisfied by the negative results of examinations and test. Often they insist that the physician order further investigative tests or prescribe something for their pain. Because there is no visible organic etiology for their complaints and because they are unsatisfied and demanding, these patients often succeed in pressuring physicians into meeting their demands. As a group they undergo many unnecessary, uncomfortable, expensive and harmful tests, during regimens and surgeries. Meanwhile, as all the examples have shown, careful, thorough and thoughtful history-taking and clinical observation are effective tools for the differential diagnosis of psychogenic pain. The secondary danger of continued treatments and tests is the reinforcement they provide for patient's beliefs that some organic cause can be found for the pain perception.

Management of all types of psychogenic pain is based on two premises: first, that analgesic, narcotic, and surgical treament of the symptom will not significantly relieve pain of psychologic origin; and second, that the underlying problem must be identified and accepted by the patient. This is usually best handled in one of the following ways:
–   confronting the patient sympathetically but directly with the fact that the pain is most likely of emotional origin;
–   recommending evaluation and treatment (psychiatric evaluation, social service counseling, antidepressant or antipsychotic medication, and so on) of the patient's emotional problem;
–   expressing willingness to continue to see the patient.

Patients are usually opposed to nonmedical management initially, and its success depends upon the ability of the primary diagnosing physician to convey sympathetic support and gain the patient's confidence. Management based upon recognition of the underlying emotional or psychological problem is more apt to be successful in relieving the secondary pain complaint. Perhaps even more importantly, this approach minimized the risk of unnecessary medical interventions, surgery, and iatrogenic drug dependence.

Suggested Reading

1   DeVaul, R.A.; Zisook, S.: Unresolved grief, clinical considerations. Postgrad. Med. *5:* 267–271 (1976).
2   DeVaul, R.A.; Zisook, S.; Stuart, J.H.: Patients with psychogenic pain. J. Fam. Prac. *4:* 53–55 (1977).
3   Engel, G.L.: Psychogenic pain and the pain-prone patient. Am. J. Med. *26:* 899–918 (1959).
4   Lindemann, E.: Symptomatology and management of acute grief. Am. J. Psych. *101:* 141–148 (1944).
5   Parkes, C.M.: Bereavement: studies of grief in adult life (International University Press, New York 1972).
6   Walters, A.: Psychogenic regional pain alias hysterical pain. Brain *84:* 1–18 (1961).
7   Zisook, S.; DeVaul, R.A.: Grief-related facsimile illness. Int. J. Psych. Med. *7:* 329–336 (1977).

Chapter VI

Other Considerations

There are several specific problems which may be discussed separately at this time. They are presented here because they apply in general to all categories of chronic pain patients.

A brief overview of some of the anatomy and physiology of pain is presented in the Appendix. However, it must be emphasized that the perception of chronic pain may or may not have anything to do with the pain pathways in any given patient. Although the majority of patients have an organic lesion which causes pain, in a chronic pain state the perception of pain very often is magnified and distorted, and it is the treatment of the abnormal perception of pain which affords the patient relief, rather than attacking the pain itself, which may not be treatable. In most patients with chronic pain, the pain pathways play only a secondary role, and numerous factors cause the pain to be magnified and perpetuated. This is in contrast to acute pain, which is the experimental model upon which these pathways have been explored.

It must be emphasized that the concept is obsolete that chronic pain can be treated by the interruption of pain pathways! This simplistic perception of chronic pain has been supplanted by the concept that the major problem in chronic pain is usually not so much the application of noxious stimulus, but magnified and distorted perception of the pain sensation and inability to cope with a painful and disabling condition. The discussion of the anatomy and physiology of some of the pain pathways is presented merely to clarify some of the concepts and rationale for management, as discussed later.

A. Narcotics and Chronic Pain

Of all of the things that are done in chronic pain clinics, probably the one which results in the greatest symptomatic improvement, when successfully concluded, is the withdrawal of pain medications. With rare exception, there is no analgesic that is effective on a long-term basis. All analgesics are designed around an acute pain model and are usually inappropriate in the chronic pain patient. Most analgesics produce tolerance within the first few weeks of use, but the side-effects persist long after. Thus, the patient is left with none of the benefits of analgesia, but all of the problems.

The side-effect which most severely perpetuates chronic pain is that of *recurrent withdrawal*. The physician provides the patient with an inappropriate medication, with no forethought about addiction or when the medication would be discontinued. The medication may be temporarily effective, but that is soon lost. By the time the effectiveness is lost, the patient is addicted and physically dependent, so if the medication is stopped, withdrawal ensues, and the patient suffers withdrawal symptoms within a few hours. The outstanding symptom of withdrawal is intensification of the patient's pain, as well as dysphoria and agitation. Both the patient and the physician feel the need to repeat the medication because of the intensification of pain. The medication 'takes the edge off the pain', not because of the analgesic properties but because it has aborted some of the withdrawal symptoms. In a few hours, the procedure is repeated. Because the withdrawal symptoms gradually become intensified, the physician feels the need to increase the dose of the medication, feeling that the pain has become more severe.

As a general rule, *there is no role in the management of chronic pain for narcotic based analgesic medications*. Such medications are useful for acute pain, when it is anticipated that they may be discontinued within a few days or weeks. Narcotics are appropriate in cancer pain, since the progressive and terminal nature of the disease outweighs considerations of addiction, even though it must be recognized that the dose must be constantly escalated as tolerance continues, sometimes to the point of oversedation, which would be totally unacceptable in a patient with chronic pain where rehabilitation is the primary goal.

Recognize that withdrawal is not something that happens only to addicts on the street who suddenly find themselves without a 'fix'. There are far more iatrogenic addicts than street addicts. Their withdrawal symptoms begin within several hours after their last dose of narcotics, so that the pattern of administration of medication and withdrawal symptoms may be repeated every 3–6 h.

Because withdrawal symptoms include agitation, depression, and impaired pain tolerance with increased pain perception, a classical pattern is set up. The patient has been taking a narcotic, for instance Percodan, one tablet four times a day for the past 6 months. He admits that the Percodan does not control his pain, but says that he takes it 'just to take the edge off'. On the other hand, when you suggest that the Percodan be discontinued, he gets extremely agitated and defensive and insists that he needs it, or may lie about the amount he takes. He tries to manipulate you into tapering it slowly (very slowly) or allowing him to taper it himself.

Let us look at a typical scenario. The patient has not had his medication for 4 h. He has become somewhat agitated and has an ill-defined feeling of distress. His pain has been getting worse over the last half hour. Because he recognizes that the medication is addicting, he tries to follow his doctor's instructions and not take it more often than every 4 h. Consequently, he is watching the clock move slowly toward the designated medication time. The pain is becoming worse. Not only is the intensity of pain perception heightened, but his tolerance to pain is decreasing rapidly, both significant manifestations of the withdrawal syndrome. Because he is so intent on the timing of his next dose of medication, he is concentrating on the intensity of the pain to assure that his next dose of medication is justified. He concentrates on the sensation to the point that it is intensified.

The momentum builds toward taking the next dose of medication. Finally, the time arrives. As the pill is swallowed, almost immediate relief ensues. (This initial relief is so effective and so prompt that it cannot be attributed to any physiologic mechanism, but illustrates the significant placebo effect.) As the medication starts to work, the patient relaxes and the pain eases. The agitation is gone, as is the heightened pain perception. The pain has become less, but will return. What has actually happened is that the narcotic withdrawal has been alleviated by the administration of the narcotic. The 'edge' is taken off the pain and the patient lies back to await the next call for medication.

This typical scene has little to do with analgesia or pain relief. It is a demonstration of the treatment of narcotic withdrawal by the administration of the same narcotic that caused the addiction. The cycle can be repeated indefinitely – withdrawal, heightened pain perception, increased pain, narcotic administration, temporary relief of both withdrawal and pain, onset of withdrawal again several hours later.

The only way to break the withdrawal cycle is to discontinue the narcotic. This means, however, that the patient may go through a period of severe narcotic withdrawal, with the attendant heightened pain perception. The rewards are worth it, but the patient must understand the reasoning and be committed to the goals of the program in order to stick with it through the period of narcotic withdrawal which may last 5 days or longer.

B. Iatrogenic Pain

It is unfortunate that much chronic pain is *iatrogenic*. Misdiagnosis and inappropriate therapy often convert a self-limited but admittedly frustrating problem into a problem which perpetuates itself because of physical or pharmacologic factors.

The patient may make the transition from a patient with an acute problem to a chronic pain patient under the eyes of his unaware physician. Sometimes it is stubborness, sometimes it is frustration, sometimes it is because the transition from an acute patient to a chronic pain patient is gradual and subtle. Yet, in many cases, early recognition that the patient is making the transition can allow a redirection of the program while the patient is still most susceptible to a chronic pain management program. This requires that both the physician and the patient understand the transition and that both accept that the program will make the adjustment from an acute interventional program to a chronic rehabilitation oriented program.

It has been said that chronic pain is an American phenomenon and occurs because patients are too free to see their physician and the physicians are too free to prescribe pain medications, many of which are promoted through Madison Avenue advertising techniques. The patient is primed through the glorified reporting of scientific achievements by the media to expect that the doctor will fix it, no matter what it is. If the doctor cannot fix it, the media tells the patient that a pill will. The patient comes to the physician with full expectation that the problem will be set straight and that the patient will have no responsibility in its management. In fact, the physician is just as subject to the influence of the media, and his expectations may be just as unrealistic. In fact, the physician may not be willing to allow the patient to take responsibility, since this may dilute the physician's feeling of authority. With such pre-existing attitudes, physician and patient may work together to develop unrealistic expectations of a treatment or medication and may over-react to the frustration of not having those unrealistic expectations fulfilled and may embark on inappropriate and self-destructive programs which may lead to chronic pain, over-medication, enforced over-restriction of activity, and perpetuation of regression and disability.

Perhaps *the most significant iatrogenic cause of chronic pain is the physician's inability, or lack of time or interest, to talk to the patient* to discover whether there are psychosocial factors distorting or intensifying the clinical picture. This is particularly important at the primary care level, since many patients go to their primary care physician not because they are feeling 'ill', but because they are feeling 'bad'. They attempt to describe their feelings in somatic terms, since that is what the physician expects. The complaints may be vague, out of proportion to the physical findings, or inconsistent with any particular problem, and yet the physician feels obligated to 'make a diagnosis'. Taking time to talk to the patient about how his symptoms are affecting his life-style or relationships may not only reveal the etiology of the symptoms, but may be therapeutic in itself.

Talking to the patient at the primary care level is the most effective prophylaxis against the development of chronic pain!

It is all too often expedient to make a snap diagnosis, order tests, or write a prescription, rather than talk to the patient to discover what he is really saying. This plants in the patient's mind the concept that he truly has a physical problem of great magnitude, which may produce a great deal of anxiety, since his primary goal in going to the physician initially may have been to seek reassurance that he was really all right. The patient then embarks on a series of negative evaluations, and ends up with anxiety added to depression. All of this, of course, intensifies the pain and perpetuates it, whether it was of psychiatric origin or a vague physical problem which could escalate readily to the classical pain syndrome.

Many patients are the victims of the 'pain reflex'. The patient walks into a doctor's office and mentions the word 'pain', and the doctor reflexly writes a prescription.

Misdiagnosis is an inevitable occurrence in the practice of medicine. Medicine is an inexact art, as well as a science, and diagnosis is very often based on assessing probabilities, rather than using absolute criteria. Misdiagnosis often leads to the failure to relieve symptoms. Even if the proper diagnosis is considered, there may not be an effective treatment available. All of these things are excusable at the present state of our art. However, the physician must be constantly on guard to detect such errors so they may be corrected. Perhaps the most common error physicians make is in locking on too firmly to an initial impression and blaming the patient if he does not respond to treatment, or, alternately, making a diagnosis for which only ineffective treatment is available and becoming impatient with the patient who does not respond. After all, it is the patient's role to get better!

One of the most common misdiagnoses concerns back and/or neck pain. What is taught in school about back and neck problems is usually taught by surgically oriented physicians. Those conditions which require surgery can usually be documented with impressive looking X-ray films or other studies. However, it is all too often left unsaid that the majority of patients with back and neck pain do not have surgical lesions, and, although their symptoms generally respond to time and appropriate management, progress may be slow and frustrating and an inconvenient restriction of activities over long periods may be necessary.

All too often the physician plays a role in perpetuating back and neck pain by (1) considering only surgical lesions in the diagnosis, (2) failing to recognize the chronic nature of the problem, or (3) failing to encourage the patient to be patient and allow sufficient time for recovery to occur. Thus, what begins as a self-limiting problem may produce permanent disability and chronic pain.

If the misdiagnosis of a surgical lesion is made, the patient may undergo a procedure that not only will not cure his symptoms, but may add additional symptoms as well. When a patient has not responded to laminectomy and fusion, the physician's response can be to blame the patient, insist that remaining symptoms are psychogenic, and start the patient on a program of escalating medications and decreasing physical activity. What is required, however, is that the physician take a new look at the patient's problem and consider whether the initial diagnosis may have been in error and whether a revision of the patient's program may be in order.

Another complicated situation arises when the physician's initial diagnosis may have been correct, but the etiology of the patient's symptoms postoperatively may not be those with which the patient initially presented. In doing any surgery, particularly surgery on the spine, it is necessary to incise and retract muscles, which may set up a new focus of myofascial injury and pain. It is common to see patients in chronic pain clinic who have undergone laminectomy considered to be a failure, but, when asked about the nature of the pain pre-operatively and postoperatively, it becomes apparent that the symptoms are quite different. Again, what is required is a reassessment of the patient's problem and embarkation on a new conservative program with acknowledgement that additional time will be required. Unfortunately, what often happens is that the patient is labeled a 'low back failure' and relegated to 'treatment by prescription', with office visits of decreasing frequency until the patient, in frustration, seeks another physician.

Even worse, both physician and patient become impatient for a cure and a second surgical procedure is performed, or even a third, fourth, or tenth or twelfth. It is acknowledged that the success rate after initial back

surgery is generally between 80 and 90%. However, after the second procedure, the success rate drops to 50% or less; after the third, it is certainly less
than 10–20%, and after the fourth, it is less than 5%. Why then do patients
end up having 6, 8 or 10 attempts at basically the same procedure? Repeat
surgery should only be considered if a specific new diagnosis is made, if it can
be documented that the original surgery was faulty, or if a specific new procedure is performed to correct the inadequacies of the original procedure.

Many patients in the Chronic Pain Clinic report that they have virtually no physical activity and, when asked why, admit that they developed
that problem while following their doctors' advice. The patient complained
of pain and the doctor's response was to tell them to limit their activity,
which is appropriate in the acute situation, but not necessarily in the
chronic. As they return to their physician week after week, each time complaining of pain, they were told each time to limit their activity even more,
until an almost complete cessation of physical activity results. The physician never took the opportunity to assess the patient's total level of physical
activity or how long the patient had been inactive, and had never thought
ahead to the possibility of remobilization.

A frequent comment by patients is 'the doctor always told me what I
could not do, but he never told me what I could do'. When a physical
condition is no longer acute, it is important to be as active as possible,
despite the symptoms, since physical inactivity and the resultant deconditioning of the musculoskeletal system later potentiates the pain.

C. Depression versus Regression

Two of the most common and interrelated complications of the
chronic pain state are regression and depression.

The large majority of patients we see at the chronic pain clinic are
regressed. They have withdrawn from normal adult physical activity and
responsibility and have frequently withdrawn from all social contacts. They
have become infantile and dependent and make little initiative in trying to
care for themselves or their families. In the patient who is overwhelmed by
life's responsibilities, or has the need to escape from the pressures of an
adult role, the regression that occurs as part of the sanction of patienthood
provides the patient with considerable primary or secondary gain. Indeed, it
is often the need to avoid such responsibilities that requires the patient to
remain in a very regressed state, and, consequently, requires the patient to

continue to have pain. It is only when the patient has established the goal of assuming more responsibility for his own welfare and rising above the regressed state that he is able to abandon sick role behavior and consequently abandon the need for his pain.

Remobilization and resocialization are designed to accomplish those goals, primarily by defeating the regression state. The patient is first required to be up and out of bed and dressed as the initial step, and later to assume more and more of the responsibility and welfare. Ultimately, the goal is for the patient to assume responsibility for others or for an occupation as well.

It is through the need for sanctioned regression that the chronic pain state is perpetuated, so that overcoming regression is an important part of management of chronic pain patients.

Although depression is less widespread in chronic pain patients, it can significantly increase pain perception and decrease pain tolerance. Much depression is the normal sequela of prolonged patienthood, that is, being disabled and/or having pain for a prolonged period of time. Much depression is secondary to the regression and to the fact that the patient is deprived of any rewarding experiences. Perhaps most important, much depression is secondary to inappropriate medications, particularly narcotic-based pain medications.

Virtually all narcotic-based pain medications have depression as a significant side effect, combined with disability and regression, which may cause profound depression. One of the important manifestations of depression is heightened pain perception and decreased pain tolerance. The pain actually feels worse, and the patient can cope with it less well.

To illustrate, consider the story of a professional football quarterback. On the first Sunday in November D.P. has been doing everything right. It is the middle of the second quarter and he has already connected for three touchdown passes. His team is ahead 21–0 and the fans and his teammates are enthusiastic and optimistic, as is he. As he takes the snap, he steps back and twists his ankle. Although it bothers him a bit, he continues to play, and, after packing the ankle in ice at halftime is able to complete the game, winning 28–7. After the game, he notices that his ankle is painful and loses time from practice over the next 3 days.

Several Sundays later, the situation is just the opposite. It is the middle of the second quarter and his team is behind 21–0. D.P. has already thrown three interceptions and has been sacked four times. Nothing is working and the fans are edgy.

On taking the ball, he steps back and twists his ankle, an identical injury to the one a few weeks earlier. He is overcome by terrible pain, and must be helped off the field. He loses the next 3 days of practice but is able to return the following week.

The injuries are identical, so what is the big difference? Pain perception is enhanced in an individual who is depressed, discouraged, and pessimistic. The same holds for the chronic pain patient as for a professional football player. It is obvious then that treatment of depression and management of discouragement are important precursors to the successful alleviation of chronic pain.

This is not to be confused with the psychogenic patient whose pain is solely a manifestation of depression. Any patient who has pain of physiologic origin has an intensification of that pain and impairment of pain tolerance if he is depressed.

Suggested Reading

1   Bausbaum, A.I.; Fields, H.L.: Endogenous pain control mechanisms. Review and hypothesis. Ann. Neurol. *4:* 451–462 (1978).
2   Dennis, S.G.; Melzack, R.: Pain-signalling systems in the dorsal and ventral spinal cord. Pain *4:* 97–132 (1977).
3   Dubner, R.: Neurophysiology of pain. Dental Clin. N. Am. *22:* 11–30 (1978).
4   Gildenberg, P.L.: Functional neurosurgery; in Schmidek, Sweet, Operative neurosurgical techniques: indications and methods (Grune & Stratton, New York 1981).
5   Mark, V.H.; Ervin, F.R.: Stereotactic surgery for relief of pain; in White, Sweet, Pain and the neurosurgeon, pp. 843–887 (Thomas, Springfield 1969).
6   Melzack, R.; Wall, P.D.: Pain mechanisms: a new theory. Science *150:* 971–979 (1965).
7   Spiegel, E.A.; Wycis, H.T.: Stereoencephalotomy. II. Clinical and physiological applications (Grune & Stratton, New York 1962).
8   Wall, P.D.: The gate theory of pain mechanisms: a re-examination and restatement. Brain *101:* 1–18 (1978).
9   Willis, W.D.; Grossman, R.G.: Medical neurobiology: neuroanatomical and neurophysiological principles basic to clinical neuroscience; 2nd ed. (Mosby, St. Louis 1977).

Chapter VII

The Doctor-Patient Relationship in Chronic Pain

Consideration of the doctor-patient relationship is a reasonable and necessary prelude for a discussion of medical management. It would be a mistake to assume that the doctor-patient relationship is any less important today than it was before the development of drugs and diagnostic and treatment procedures of the last several decades. In chronic pain or illness, this relationship takes on even greater significance. To understand why, it is necessary to know something about the expectations that patients and physicians bring to their relationship.

Three different sets of expectations influence the doctor-patient relationship. They are the learned social role expectation, the fantasied or wishful expectations and, lastly, those expectations which correspond most closely to the situation at hand and its possible real outcomes.

Role, in the present sense, refers to a set of expectations that defines one's position in the social structure. The expectations are culturally determined and unconsciously accepted by those assuming the role. They are almost exclusively implied rather than stated. For example, the social expectation in western civilized society that adults wear clothing while going about daily public business is not open to individual interpretation nor subject to debate, and not overtly stated to those who assume the role 'sane adult'. A set of unconsciously learned expectations defines the social role 'sick' also. *Talcott Parsons,* probably the best known medical sociologist, detailed the role expectations of the doctor-patient interaction for the first time in 1951 (table II). He says first that, because of their illness or disability, the sick are relieved of certain social obligations. From the viewpoint of society, not carrying out one's obligations is undesirable or deviant behavior, so the sick role is a deviant role. But, unlike the healthy who are held accountable for inadequate social role performance, the sick are forgiven their inferior performance and considered not responsible for their deviant status, i.e., for having become ill. This is the primary 'privilege' of patienthood – temporary exemption from normal responsibilities.

Table II. Privileges and obligations of the roles of physicians, healthy adults, and acute patients

	Status	Privileges	Obligations
Physician	responsible	professional prestige; authority	professional competence; availability; caring for patient; placing patient's welfare foremost
Healthy adult	responsible	personal, bodily integrity and autonomy	role fulfillment, e.g., breadwinner, spouse, parent, church member, etc.
Acute patient	not responsible	exemption from social responsibility; entitled to be taken care of (child-like behavior encouraged)	desire to leave sick role; effort to seek professional help; compliance with professional advice; loss of autonomy

A second privilege of the sick role is the occupant's right to be taken care of. This right frequently results in the patient's adoption of a more dependent, child-like manner (regressing). Another consequence of the right to be cared for is that the patient accepts neither the responsibility for the illness nor the reponsibility for treating it, both of which are now seen as the physician's problems.

The sick role has its set of responsibilities also. The primary responsibility of the new role ordinarily is that the occupant desires to return to health and the resumption of former duties. This generates two more obligations – the obligation to seek professional help and the obligation to comply with the advice and instruction of the physician or healthy professional. Social sick role expectations are so firmly established that hospital staff members often react with anger when they think a patient is not cooperating or does not want to get well. There is a notable lack of curiosity about a patient's reasons for not wanting to get well and little tolerance for the dying patient who cannot get well. Much psychiatric consultation on medical services is initiated because an uncooperative patient does not seem to want to, or cannot get well.

The sick role, then, is a legitimate way to be excused from adult responsibilities and to become child-like again. Because society needs to limit its number of non-contributing members, physicians perform the important social function of controlling admission to the sick role. Their function is institutionalized in such procedures as requiring a physician's excuse to miss work and requesting his judgments concerning disability and competency to stand trial. These judgments provide the only socially sanctioned exemptions from adult responsibility and are therefore very powerful. When this exemption is sought after, consciously or unconsciously, much dedication and perseverance can be brought to the search.

Beyond their function of legitimizing sick role occupancy, physicians' obligations, according to *Parsons,* are essentially two-fold. They are expected to place patient interests and well-being above their own, and they are expected to care for the patient in a concerned and professionally competent way. On the practical level, putting patient interests foremost means availability and a professional approach to medicine. It is tempting to speculate that these social expectations are the basis for the major political issues currently surrounding health care delivery. Perhaps what is being considered the lack or maldistribution of physicians is, in part patient perception that physicians ar not immediately available to them. Patients translate their social 'right' to be taken care of into expectations that every physician be available to every patient at every moment.[1]

The second major expectation of doctors is that they care for their patients in a professionally competent way. This demands that they be sympathetic and understanding to the person, besides being interested in the illness. Also, however, it means that they do not become so involved with patients emotionally as to jeopardize good medical judgment. Finally, it assumes that physicians will bring competence in diagnostic and treatment skills to the task.

These social role expectations for physician and patient are powerful determinants of behavior. When a person visits a doctor's office, both sets of role expectations begin to operate. Physicians conduct the interview and

---

[1] Although such expectations are unrealistic, it is not impossible to maintain a critical degree of availability. For example, during my psychiatry residency (*R.A.D.*) and in my general practice I encouraged patients to call me at any time. I was available to them 24 hours a day. With this assurance, my patients almost never called; in fact, they protected me, because I was 'such a good doctor'. Some colleagues took the opposite tack and, deluged with complaints from dependent, overdemanding patients, got unlisted phone numbers which made it more difficult for their patients to reach them. The apprehension and anxiety this induced led to extreme, often successful, attempts on the part of patients to track them down.

examination with the unspoken assumption that the individual has a medical problem. The patient-to-be expects the problem to be named and a treatment program planned. The physician who decides after evaluation that there is no organic disease process in operation and informs the patient of this decision violates the implicit understanding that the patient is sick and the doctor will diagnose and treat the illness. Not being able to fulfill patients' expectations may arouse in the physician a need to compensate for the role violation, perhaps by prescribing harmless (or not so harmless) drugs. This further confuses patients who sense that the doctor does not have a firm idea of what is wrong, but know they are sick and need medication. Prescribing inappropirate drugs is also counter-productive in the many cases of patients whose visits are occasioned by complaints that are the result of the stresses of living. The drugs often induce secondary depression and addiction. At the very least, they can be expected to foster psychological regression.

Equally powerful are the *fantasized role expectations* brought to the doctor-patient relationship. These are less well understood and much more individual than the social expectations. They arise in part from a practical necessity of medical intervention. Patients must allow physicians to undertake invasive, oftentimes painful, procedures. In order to do so, they must be willing to hand over management of their health to an outsider. Regressive child-like behavior that accompanies sick role occupancy makes this transfer of responsibility easier, but the patient must be emotionally able to effect the transfer. The fantasied or wishful expectations of the doctor-patient relationship help establish the necessary emotional climate. The first such fantasy is the patient's wish for a magical parent perceived as all-knowing and all-caring. Few of us who have been seriously ill are unaware of the overpowering desire to turn ourselves over to someone we trust and someone we believe to be omnipotent. The presence of this fantasy allows patients to satisfy a sick role requirement, namely, placing responsibility for their well-being in the hands of the physician. This transfer of power can be of critical importance if acute medical intervention is necessary.

A second and equally active fantasy is that one will be treated in the way one has been treated during past illness. This is a complex wish in which the meanings of the caretakers and the fact of being cared for are often more significant than what actually occurred during the illness. Patient desires to repeat a past experience with illness can result in repetitive patterns of difficulty with doctors; patterns which are both understandable in the context of the medical histories and strong predictors of present and future illness behavior. One adolescent patient, for example refused to accept the fact that she had ulcerative colitis and had left four hospitals against medical advice prior to her admission to our teaching hospital. In each instance she had appeared at first to be a cooperative and interesting patient and had elicited more than average attention from nurses and doctors. At the point where she was expected to become involved in the management of her own illness, on each occasion she suddenly refused to cooperate and signed out against medical advice. This history predicted that the same behavior would occur until a major intervention interrupted the pattern of response.

Recognizing that patients wish to be treated as they have in the past means recognizing also the importance of inquiring carefully into their medical histories and experiences in the sick role. Replies to such inquiries help the physician understand what illness means to the patient and give evidence of a patterned response to medical intervention. In both types of fantasied expectations – the wish for a magical caretaker and the wish to repeat past illness experience – the model for the medical professional is usually the parents or other important caretakers, making these two aspects of child-like relationship to the physician, components of what is called *transference* in psychotherapy.

Rather than recognizing the fantasy expectations as sources of information and means to facilitate physician intervention, physicians run the risk of believing that they should be able to meet the unrealistic expectations. Pressure also stems from the unstated social role expectations that physicians name and treat illness. They want, therefore, to fulfill their role obligations, as they see them, and to satisfy patient expectations. Patients' needs for physicians to be omnipotent and omnificent magical parents oftentimes coincides with physicians' needs to be bigger than life. In the face of the incessant demands and inherent uncertainties of medical practice, it is tempting to suppose that one can be the all-knowing and all-powerful parent.

The wishes and fantasied expectations of the patient can be discussed at the beginning of the medical workup and, in fact, such questions as: 'What do you think is wrong' and 'What do you think would make you well?' may elicit useful information. Any overt or covert acknowledgement, however, that the patient's expectations are going to be met is premature and unwise. Medical experience teaches that unusual or unrealistic expectations on the part of physician or patient, or both, frequently lead to frustration and disappointment at the end of a negative workup.

The medical task is to apply professional skills in the patient's best interest. An awareness of both social role expectations and personal, fantasied expectations aid in the execution of medical management, since very few medical situtations are of the strictly physiological, fractured leg variety. Although patients may complain to the physician of physical discomfort, in a majority of cases non-somatic concern – often anxiety, stress or loss – lead people to consult physicians. Age and sex, along with psychological, social cultural and ethnic factors, play a part in the decision to seek medical help. Presence of frank medical signs and symptoms not only ranks low on the list of reasons for consulting a physician, but may even lead to delay in seeking medical consultation. This can be especially true if the symptoms are associated in the patient's mind with serious threat to health or life. Beware, however; so thorough is the human defense mechanism of denial that patients who apologize to the doctor for their presence, saying they are just going through a difficult time, very often have underlying medical illness. At the other end of a continuum are those who insist they have serious medical illness which demands immediate diagnosis and treatment and who, in all likelihood, are suffering from anxiety.

The first part of the physician's task, then, is to find out specifically why the patient is there and what expectations (fantasied, social and realistic) he or she entertains about the present interaction. Again a thorough, thoughtful history-taking should provide most of this information. Beyond the facts of past injuries, illness, hospitalizations and surgeries, history-taking should get at some details of the patient's social background and present circumstances, family and family deaths, and feelings about past experiences with illness. Patients might be asked how they interpret the symptoms they describe and also how the present symptoms interfere with their established way of life. Again, any assumption at this point in the evaluation that the patient has an acute illness, any granting of sick-role status, or any covert assurance that the patient's expectations will be fulfilled is not only premature but is a threat to the therapeutic potential of the doctor-patient relationship.

Clues gained from history-taking usually indicate how the examination should proceed. It is important here that patient and physician understand and agree on how the complaint is to be evaluated further, that is, whether physical examination, tests or X-rays or, perhaps, psychiatric assessment is desirable. The types of interventions physicians are finally called upon to make can be broadly classified as administrative, acute medical, or chronic interventions.

Requests for *administrative intervention* are common in primary care practice. They may be overt, as when a physician's permission to miss or return to work is required. They may be covert, as when the 'patient' is really seeking disability status, compensation eligibility, or exemption from military service. Patients at the anxiety end of the continuum may be looking for sanctioned sick-role occupancy as a way to avoid stressful adult responsibilities. In such cases, and where the primary care physicians do not feel competent to help these patients uncover underlying problems, they should be able to suggest sources for social or psychiatric intervention.

Often patients, reluctant to state their administrative requests, arrive at clinics and doctors' offices with physical complaints, expecting physicians, as magical parents, to guess and provide what they are really seeking. Family concerns, such as a desire for help in placing an aged parent in a nursing home or in dealing with an alcoholic member, may occasion this sort of clinical situation.

An example will illustrate the non-medical range of such requests. Medical evaluation of a patient who complained of vague abdominal discomfort revealed symptoms suggestive of possible gastritis and heavy alcohol intake. A medical investigative plan was outlined and counsel was given for dealing with the drinking problem. When the patient refused further evaluation, a psychiatrist was called in and ascertained that the patient had come to the outpatient clinic hoping that the physician would contact his spouse whom his drinking had estranged. Once the request was identified, the patient was assisted in arranging for marital counseling and, this accomplished, he was willing to proceed with the medical evaluation. Clearly, assuming acute illness and activating acute medical intervention would not be in the best interest of the patient who has need for administrative services.

The proper role of *acute medical intervention* needs little elaboration because it is the model in which physicians are trained. Interactions between the doctor and the acutely ill patient fit social sick-role theory best. The patient's position can be symoblized by a formula that represents two important aspects of sick role status. The most dramatic example of a person in this position is the comatose or unconscious patient, but the classification includes all those suffering from acute infectious processes, trauma, injury, cardiovascular accident and stroke, and acute exacerbations of chronic disease.

Because the social role expectations match more closely with what can realistically be expected from the medical task at hand, less patient dissatisfaction or physician frustration is expected in acute medical situations. Fantasied expectations can still interfere, in the ways described earlier, however, unless they are recognized and managed.

It is most important to remember that the acute intervention role of the physician is only temporary. As the acute crisis passes and the patient moves toward either former health or an adjusted normal status with some disability, the roles of doctor and patient must change. The classic example of the diabetic patient illustrates the process clearly. The diagnosis of diabetes is frequently made under acute clinical conditions – someone brought to the hospital with a diabetic complication or in coma. The physician takes on responsibility for the patient's illness, makes a diagnosis and reestablishes normal physiological balance in the patient. At this point the roles must begin to change and the patient must assume responsibility for long-term management.

As *Szasz and Hollender* point out, the physician must be the first to recognize and adjust to the changing needs of the patient. The acutely ill are disabled but accept no responsibility for their own care. Patients with chronic illness must accept emotionally that they have an incurable problem and that the responsibility for its management is principally theirs. Their task then is to overcome or minimize disability from the disorder.

There are at least three non-medical reasons why this is difficult to achieve. First, aggressive independent self-management violates social sick role expectation. Secondly, such behavior leaves fantasied wishes for magical parent care unsatisfied. Thirdly, much description of illness behavior in the past and most medical literature saw the 'sick person' as the *acutely* sick person, and ignored the description of well-adjusted patients with chronic illness. More recently, physicians and sociologists have recognized the need to address chronic illness as a separate issue and a literature is beginning to accumulate on chronic pain management.

Let us return to the diabetic patient, still hospitalized and with normal physiological balance recently restored. The medical task at this point becomes an educational task. Ideally, the physician defines the illness, outlines a management plan and allows the patient to take on as much responsibility for treatment and management as possible. As the patient improves, he or she accepts responsibility for the incurable disease, gains experience in diet planning and urine sugar measurement, learns to administer insulin, and may become as knowledgeable about diabetes as the physician. The physician becomes passive, serving as a counselor or partner in the management. There is evidence that physicians are poor at educating patients to accept and manage their illnesses. Poor compliance with chronic illness management regimens suggests that patients do not understand their illnesses and still view the physician as being responsible for managing them.

The chief responsibility of those who occupy the chronic sick role is to work toward minimizing disability and establishing an adjusted normal role for themselves. Many medical and social problems obstruct attainment of this goal. First, the illness may cause limitations or alterations of former life style. A less obvious hindrance is the dependency and regression that accompany the disabled role. It is never easy for the chronic patient to give up the privileges of the sick role and the comfort of being cared for. Reassuming adult responsibilities can be even more difficult. All the psychological, social, cultural, and ethnic factors that affect patient's decisions to assume the sick role affect also their willingness or reluctance to leave it. Reluctance to leave the sick role, 'disability from being disabled', and disability from the illness can blend together in the patient's mind. If this is the case, the physician, in the new chronic intervention role, might help the patient sort out the causes and extent of disability, or suggest someone or some group which can.

Family dynamics can hinder the patient's return to the adjusted normal role. Caring for the patient can give meaning to a family member's role, or, if a powerful member is ill, others may enjoy new independence and decision-making. In both cases, sincere family support for the sick member's recovery is compromised by the benefit other family members receive from the disability situation.

Social and legal stipulations for return to work which specify 'complete recovery' can frustrate the patient's attempts to assume an adjusted normal role. Physicians are called upon to legitimize return to the role 'healthy adult' just as they are used to legitimize 'sick adult'. They are reluctant to declare someone completely recovered who is still somewhat regressed and has not resumed normal activity; that is, someone who is still disabled by the sick role. On the other hand, the patient will never recover fully until he or she can return to social responsibility, at least partially. Compensation and litigation factors cause similar legal entanglements from which it becomes increasingly difficult for the disabled to escape.

Experience in the chronic pain service has led us to believe that an understanding of the personal and social role expectations of the doctor-patient relationship are critical to constructive intervention. Either or both sets of expectations can prejudice assessment of a patient complaint. Physicians, as subject to the pressure of these expectations as their patients, must not assume, or give patients cause to infer, that social and fantasied expectations for acute care will be met. Instead, they must attempt to determine the true nature of the complaint and their patient's underlying reasons for seeking medical help at that particular time.

Patients' real needs may range from a desire for administrative services to a need for acute care or for help in the management of a chronic problem. Social and personal expectations and physician training often make it difficult for physicians to recognize and act upon the last of these – the need for chronic care intervention. Much of the remainder of this volume will deal with just those interventions.

If the patient fails to make the transition to a state of adjustment to chronic disability, he often becomes a 'chronic pain patient'.

Suggested Reading

1   Bird, B.: Talking with patients (Lippincott, Philadelphia 1955).
2   DeVaul, R.A.; Faillace, L.A.: Persistent pain and illness insistence. Am. J. Surg. *135:* 828–833 (1978).
3   DeVaul, R.A.; Zisook, S.: Chronic pain syndromes: the psychiatrist's role. Psychosomatics *19:* 417–421 (1978).
4   Fordyce, W.E.; Fowler, R.S., Jr.; Lehmann, J.F.; LeLateur, B.J.; Sand, P.L.; Trieschmann, R.B.: Operant conditioning in the treatment of chronic pain. Archs phys. Med. Rehabil. *54:* 399–408 (1973).
5   Mechanic, D.: The concept of illness behavior. J. chron. Dis. *15:* 189–194 (1961).
6   Parsons, T.: The social system, pp. 428–479 (Free Press, New York 1951).
7   Szasz, T.S.; Hollender, M.H.: A contribution to the philosophy of medicine: the basic models of doctor-patient relationship. Archs intern. Med. *97:* 585–592 (1956).

Chapter VIII

Evaluation

This chapter concerns the evaluation of the chronic pain patient by history and physical examination. The first step in evaluating a patient with chronic pain is the recognition that the patient has chronic pain. This is easy for those who see a patient on referral to a chronic pain center, since the act of referral in itself tends to designate the patient as a chronic pain patient. When, on the other hand, a physician has followed a patient day-to-day, has struggled with the patient through a multitude of unsuccessful treatments, and has witnessed the gradual deterioration of the patient, it is not easy for this physician to decide one day that the patient no longer fits the pattern upon which all prior treatment was based but has progressed to a new category, that of 'chronic pain patient', for which the management is markedly different.

This is an especially difficult decision when the physician becomes close to his patient. It is difficult to ask a friend, 'What underlying psychological stresses do you have that may be contributing to your disability?' It is even more difficult for the friend to reply objectively. Likewise, it is particularly difficult for the physician who may have operated on the patient initially to concede failure and recognize even that perhaps the surgery should not have been done in the first place.

Every physician has difficulty recognizing that the reason a patient does not respond to specific treatment is that, under his very eyes, the patient has become a chronic pain patient with a need for a more comprehensive program. Yet, it is those physicians who find themselves in precisely these situations who must determine that the patient has become a chronic pain patient and change the direction of the treatment program completely.

We have attended many conferences in which selection of patients for various pain-relieving procedures was discussed. With great regularity, an erudite discussion of criteria for including patients in any treatment program concludes with a statement such as, 'After I have tested the patient with all of the above techniques, I find that the most reliable index of success of treatment is the "gut reaction" that I get about the patient.' No matter how elaborate or sophisticated a program has been developed for predicting success in treatment of pain patients, the 'gut reaction' seems to be the most reliable for many perceptive physicians.

All of the formulae and reasoned discourse in the world do not take the place of empathy which, fortunately, most physicians have innately and which, unfortunately, other physicians are never able to acquire. The evaluation of chronic pain patients does not require a specialist in psychiatry, neurosurgery, anesthesiology, or pain, but rather an empathetic and observant evaluator who has a feeling for the simple dynamics of interpersonal daily living.

With that in mind, we can only advise the obvious 'listen to your patient'. He will tell you something if you take the time to listen and the effort to encourage him. He may talk of 'pain' and mean 'distress' or 'suffering'. He may put psychological complaints into somatic terms, either because he perceives them more concretely in that fashion or because he can speak of them more readily to you in that fashion. Many a patient goes to his doctor saying, 'I have pain,' when he is really saying, 'I am suffering and need help but don't know how to ask for it.'

A. History

Perhaps the most useful diagnostic tool is listening carefully to the patient's description of his pain, asking questions about his activities and his ideas about his pain problem, observing his actions throughout the interview and examination, and talking with his accompanying spouse or caretaker to obtain a comprehensive clinical history. By the end of the interview, the doctor should be able to imagine exactly what the patient feels and what the patient is really calling 'pain'. Considerable attention should be given to evaluating the patient's disability as well as his pain, since treatment often may be directed to the disability rather than the primary complaint itself.

The patient should have the opportunity to describe his pain in detail. Beware of patients whose descriptions are too vague or too elaborate. The patient who is unable to describe his pain may have only the vaguest concept of what pain is, and may be referring to distress rather than to physical pain. The patient whose description is so elaborate and detailed that the pain defies anatomical or physiological explanation may be concentrating on his pain so greatly that it is blown out of proportion.

It is important not to lead the patient, for frequently the patient's description will coincide little with the examiner's preconceived notion. The simple initial question, 'What brings you here today?,' or the simple directive, 'Tell me about your symptoms,' may evoke revealing and rewarding answers.

Patients use many terms to describe their pain, and there are several elaborate protocols for listing and evaluating those terms. However, in the usual office setting, it is sufficient merely to ask the patient to describe his pain (table III). After the patient's spontaneous description, considerable additional information can be obtained by asking specifics.

What is the *character* of the pain? It is sharp or dull? Is it aching or burning? What does the pain feel like? It's like a muscle cramp. 'It's like someone standing on my foot.' 'It's like a toothache.' 'It's like an electric shock.' Overly dramatic descriptors may indicate excessive emotional involvement in the pain process – 'It's like an elephant standing on my foot.' 'It's like a thousand nails being driven into my hand.' Particularly revealing may be, 'This is just like the pain my wife had before she died of cancer.'

Disagreeable sensations may not involve the pain pathways per se, even though the patient may call them pain. Unless the patient describes what is classically pain, procedures involving interruption or stimulation of the pain pathways are of little benefit. Patients may describe their pain as a pulling or pressure sensation not defined clinically as pain. The patient with a rectal malignancy may describe his pain as, 'It feels like I'm sitting on a rock,' or 'It always feels like I have to move my bowels.' These describe visceral sensations which are not carried via the classical pain pathways.

In the description of the *intensity* of the patient's pain, it is necessary to have more than just a description such as 'severe' or 'unbearable'. How does the pain interfere with the patient's activities? The patient who describes 'unbearable' pain may tell of participating in activities and hobbies which such severe pain would preclude. The patient may describe his pain as not being particularly severe, but he may be totally and inappropriately disabled from it.

The next question concerns the *distribution* of the pain. Description of a radicular pattern of pain may be helpful in determining the etiology. The initial description of the pain distribution may be incomplete or misleading. If he complains of back pain, is it really at the site of a prior laminectomy or has it now changed to the renal area? Is leg pain truly in a radicular distribution or might it be hip pain? In most cases, it is helpful to ask the patient to describe the back pain and the leg pain separately, whereupon it might be

Table III. History

I.   The patient's general description of the pain
    A. Character of the pain
    B. Intensity of the pain
    C. Distribution of the pain
    D. Activities which increase/decrease pain
    E. Narcotic use and recurrent withdrawal
    F. Origin of this pain
        1. When
        2. How
    G. Prior treatments for this pain and response to each
    H. What do you think is wrong?
    I. What do you think would make you well?
II.   Family history
    A. Diseases
    B. Pain problems
    C. Surgeries
    D. Family deaths and patient's reaction
III.   Social history
    A. Former responsibilities
    B. Former hobbies/sports
    C. Activity profile at present
        1. How much time is spent in bed?
        2. Does patient require care from another?
        3. What activities/hobbies does patient engage in?
    D. Proposed activities if pain were alleviated
    E. Pending litigation/compensation
IV.   Past medical history
    A. Childhood illness
    B. Prior illness or injury and response to treatment
    C. Feelings about past experiences with illness
V.   Interview with spouse/caretaker

discovered that these two pains are unrelated. It is surprising how often patients who have had several unsuccessful laminectomies may be complaining of a disabling pain involving the muscles of the back, with only minor occasional leg pain, much of which may be referred. Close examination or trigger point blocks may indicate a myofascial syndrome which can be treated locally, rather than a recurrent disc problem which might require further studies.

The physician should inquire what makes the pain *worse*. This may reveal a mechanical cause for the pain, which may in turn suggest a course of treatment. Is there any particular motion that makes the pain worse? Is there any particular position that provokes the pain? It is particularly important to note if there are emotional factors which make the pain worse, such as, 'The pain gets worse when I'm nervous.' Especially revealing might be, 'The pain gets worse when I try to have intercourse, so we just don't do that anymore.' If there are episodes of the pain becoming worse, do they follow any particular pattern? Do the acute exacerbations occur at the same time of year. If so, is it the anniversary of some emotion-laden event such as the death of a loved one? Do the episodes coincide with weekends or vacation time, or visits from any particular relatives?

What makes the pain *better?* Again, answers may suggest possible treatment. Is the pain better when the patient lies down? If so, is there any particular position of comfort? Is the pain better with local application of heat? Is it better with local application of cold? What treatments may have afforded partial relief in the past?

Pain that is not altered by physical factors, such as lying down or usual physical activities, is not likely to be of mechanical etiology, nor are physical treatments likely to help. Pain that remains constant 'no matter what' is very often of psychogenic etiology.

It should be recognized that many patients experience temporary relief, usually 6–12 weeks, after unsuccessful surgery. This should not be interpreted as being encouraging as far as long-term relief is concerned, since it is a consistent pattern in therapeutic failures. Consequently, no procedure for the relief of pain should be evaluated prior to 3–6 months, since late recurrences during that time are so common.

One must be particularly careful in trying to evaluate the effectiveness of analgesic medication. Keeping in mind that no analgesic is without both tolerance and addiction over the long term, and no analgesic medication is effective against chronic pain, the physician might recognize the typical pattern of recurrent withdrawal. The patient reports that his Percodan (or Darvon, etc.) 'doesn't really get rid of the pain, but it takes the edge off'. When it is suggested that the medication be discontinued, a typical response is that the patient must have it in case he has severe pain, even though admittedly the medication is not effective. Indeed, the patient may become agitated or hostile if it is insisted too strongly without explanation that he do without his medication.

When did the pain *begin?* It may be found that the patient actually had some pain prior to an accident. The pain may have begun spontaneously on the anniversary of the death of a family member. The pain may have begun the day after divorce proceedings were begun, or during an equally stressful time of life.

How did the pain *begin?* Was the onset gradual or abrupt? Was the onset coincident with trauma or illness? Did the pain appear gradually over many weeks? If the patient has a history of an accident, were the trauma and the onset of symptoms really temporally related?

If the patient has an involved history of *prior treatments,* particularly surgery, it is important to know what symptoms the patient had going into the treatment and what symptoms the patient had coming out. It should *not* be assumed that the patient's surgery was for the same pain that now brings him to the doctor, nor that the diagnosis that prompted prior surgery was necessarily accurate.

One extremely common pattern which is often unrecognized, and is heretofore unreported, involves the patient who has had a laminectomy for classic lumbar radiculopathy presenting with both back and leg pain. Following surgery, the leg pain goes away or changes, but the back pain remains. The back pain may be intensified or, frequently, changed in character. When the patient returns to say that he still has pain, the physician assumes it is the same pain he had prior to surgery. Actually it may be the pain of a local myofascial syndrome. Such myofascial pain, resulting from a local injury to muscle and/or tendon secondary to muscle resection and retraction that occurred with the laminectomy may respond to a local program of trigger point injections, physical therapy, and muscle stretching exercises.

It is often interesting to ask the patient what he thinks is wrong. Frequently the patient will take a very mechanistic attitude towards his pain complaint. He may picture bones rubbing against each other, adhesions strangulating bowel, nerve being pinched vise-like by boney protuberances, or rampaging cancer where none exists.

Often the chronic pain patient is one who demands an explanation for every body symptom, including those which are normal physiologic sensations. Unfortunately, too many physicians feel compelled to explain every sensation, even when an explanation is not known or justified, and the patient's various physicians may give various explanations. This often serves to perpetuate the patient's conviction that something significant is wrong and, at the same time, to perpetuate the chronic pain.

A *family history,* with greater detail than usual about illnesses which have familial predisposition, may be quite revealing. The physician should inquire about chronic pain or symptoms of pain associated with serious illness of other family members. It is not uncommon for a patient to identify with an ill or deceased loved one. Fear of a fatal illness may intensify symptoms or the patient may assume the symptoms of a deceased family member for whom he was unable to grieve.

The *social history* is of interest. Particularly important are those factors which revolve around not only the patients's pain but also his disability. What was the patient able to do prior to the pain; what can he no longer do? How important are these activities to him? What personal, family and social obligations is the patient no longer able to bear?

What is the patient's *activity profile?* Ask the patient to describe an average day. What time does he wake up? What does he do after he wakes up? How much of the day does he remain out of bed? Conversely, does he return to bed during the day, and, if so, for how long? What does he do for diversion? What social activities does the patient have? What hobbies does the patient have?

Is the patient independent or does he require care? Is the amount of care that the patient receives appropriate to the objective evidence of physical disability, or is it in excess of that, that is, does the patient receive excessive secondary gain from the complaint of pain?

It is interesting to ask the patient what he would do if the pain were suddenly relieved. Patients whose answers show that they have not thought realistically of this possibility may have already decided that their pain will not be relieved despite any or all treatment. It is advisable to consider practical goals for treatment early in the program, but asking about the patient's own goals prior to this might indicate whether he has a realistic understanding of his problem.

Of great importance in a pain patient's history are facts concerning *litigation and compensation.* Some physicians shy away from questioning in this area, feeling that they would be encroaching on the patient's privacy or that these questions are not fair. However, financial considerations are often paramount in the perpetuation of the patient's pain and should be investigated. Although often unsaid, it must be recognized that if a patient loses his pain while litigation is in process, the loss may significantly and adversely affect the award. At the end of the two to three years necessary for a disability case to go successfully through the court (and perhaps more than that, if appeals are involved), the patient may be irreversibly disabled, addicted, immobilized, and thoroughly conditioned to have pain. If the pain is the result of a job-related injury, it is important, both from the legal and clinical standpoints, to obtain a detailed history about the mechanism of injury and the relationship of the injury to the patient's chronic pain complaint.

The *past medical history* is of considerable importance as well. Not only may certain factors have predisposed the patient to injury or illness, but the groundwork may have been laid for the patient's chronic pain behavior. What was the patient's response to illness or injury in the past? Has the patient an inordinate number of episodes of disability?

Many people are so predisposed to chronic pain that they can be considered chronic pain patients waiting for an opportunity to express themselves.

The physician should inquire about those characteristics outlined in the discussion of the typical chronic pain patient (q.v.). Does the patient have a history of childhood illnesses? Did the patient come from a large family and receive secondary gain, attention, and relief from responsibility through childhood illnesses? Were there other chronic pain problems in the past? Did the patient tend to be 'sickly'? How many surgeries has the patient had? What presenting symptom led to each surgery; were the illnesses those that are classically associated with objective physical findings or with subjective complaints, principally pain? What was the time of the surgeries, particularly in regard to the developmental years? How many operations were performed because of failure of prior surgery or failure of conservative management?

Ideally, the history should be taken with the patient alone and again with the *spouse* or *caretaker* present and the two interviews contrasted. Sometimes spouses' promotion of the pain is evident in their answering for the patient or filling in dramatic details of bodily sensation that only the patient could perceive. The patient may report relatively modest pain, but the spouse embellishes the complaint to make it appear more dramatic. The spouse may hurry to assist the patient in even the most minor activities, not allowing the patient to do anything at all for himself. It is obvious how such behavior promotes dependency and regression. Where this is observed, interviewing the spouse may give some insight into the spouse's need for the patient to be regressed and dependent. A complementary situation – one in which a patient wants to be dependent and a spouse needs the patient to be dependent – promotes pain behavior so strongly that treatment may be to no avail. For this reason, it is important to include the spouse in counseling and in the patient's program.

In summary, the history should be detailed. It should solicit sufficient information about the pain so that the physician can appreciate precisely the sensation about which the patient complains. It should contain questions about pain behavior and pain perception as well as about the pain per se. It should attempt to identify those characteristics which are described elsewhere as typical characteristics of chronic pain patients. It should review how the pain affects the patient's life and how factors in the patient's life may affect the pain.

It is only when the psychological, social, and physical factors are considered together that some insight into the many facets of chronic pain can be obtained, and it is only by considering these many facets that a comprehensive and effective chronic pain treatment program can be designed.

B. Physical Examination

Physical examination of the patient with chronic pain should be carried out with the same thoroughness brought to the examination of any other new patient (table IV). It should include a search for underlying etiologies regardless of previous diagnoses. Remember that although proffered histories and reports can be helpful, they can also be very misleading. There is a tendency to label a patient fairly early in his clinical career and everafter select only those tests intended to verify the initial diagnosis. When a patient presents with chronic pain, it is often helpful to take a fresh look at the patient's problem, remembering also that not all problems are related. For instance, it is not uncommon for a patient who has been appropriately treated for lumbar radiculopathy to present later with back pain of muscular origin. Even when a patient has had a diagnosis of cancer in the past, all new problems may not be due to metastatic disease.

If the patient brings previous X-rays and laboratory studies with him, the physician should examine the films directly and not rely only on the written reports. Remember that the patient is presenting with chronic pain because he did not respond to treatment of the originally diagnosed condition, so that original diagnosis should be reassessed each time the patient is evaluated.

Chronic pain patients have a high incidence of *undiagnosed medical problems unrelated to their chief complaint*. The pain complaint often becomes so great a focus of attention that other complaints are either unreported or overlooked. Significant unrelated medical illness very often co-exists with chronic pain. In our experience, nearly a quarter of the patients who report to a chronic pain clinic have unrelated medical problems, some

Table IV. Physical examination

I.   General examination
     A. Physical problems unrelated to pain symptom
     B. Physical problems related to pain symptom
         1. Observation of patient's general demeanor
         2. Observation of patient when he is 'unobserved'
         3. Comparison of mobility with description of disability
         4. Notice of inappropriate responses

II. Validity of findings
     A. Hysterical pain and malingering
     B. Sensory examination
     C. Motor examination

III. Examination of the pain complaint
     A. General approach to examination of any painful area
         1. Distribution of the pain
         2. Appearance of the painful area
         3. Palpation of muscle
         4. Manipulation of the body part
     B. Considerations in musculoskeletal pain
         1. Myofascial syndrome
         2. Low back pain
         3. Trigger blocks
     C. Other diagnostic blocks

---

of which, such as heart disease, syphilis, tuberculosis, or collagen disease, are quite serious.

One must be particularly wary of missing medical problems in this group of patients for several reasons. First, the patient's entire attention is directed to his chief complaint, chronic pain. His pain becomes all-consuming and the center of all his attention, so that other symptoms may not arouse sufficient concern. Second, the symptoms of the unrelated condition may be interpreted as being part of the primary pain complaint. It is not unusual for the physician to miss the significance of the left arm pain in a patient who complains of multiple pains throughout the body, particularly if those pains already involve the cervical area or upper extremities. Third, considerable debility accompanies the disabled, regressed state in which many pain patients find themselves. The polypharmacy associated with management of chronic pain patients might either provoke an illness as a side-effect, or the side-effects of the drug may mask such an illness. Fourth, patients with chronic pain may report their symptoms inaccurately, since such reports are colored by their own somatic preoccupation. Finally, the physician may not attach sufficient significance to the complaint of a patient when the complaint is one of a long series of unrelated undiagnosed complaints. Remember, even 'crocks' get sick!

The reports of pain and tenderness, restricted activity, or other subjective reports generated as part of the patient's physical examination may be misleading, so that the physician must rely more critically on objective criteria. This approach has been described not inaccurately as a veterinary medicine approach to the physical examination.

It is often advantageous to leave examination of the patient's chief complaint until the end of the general physical examination. Many patients will become so involved in reporting distress when they are being examined for their chronic pain that there is considerable spill-over into the general physical examination as well, intensifying the inaccuracy of the reporting. It should, however, be explained that the general examination will be done first, so the patient does not feel obligated to register his complaints prematurely. The general examination is, for the most part, the same as that for any patient with a medical complaint, so its specifics will not be detailed here.

Observations of the patient's demeanor during the general part of the physical examination, however, may take on added significance and should be compared and contrasted with the patient's demeanor during that part of the examination directed to the chief complaint. An abrupt change in the patient's personality or attitude may signify excessive emotional involvement in the chief complaint.

Physical problems related to the pain symptom should be evaluated at the conclusion of the general physical examination. The physical examination is an opportunity to observe and talk to the patient at a time when attention is not directed to the history of his complaint. Accompanying the patient down the hall to the examining room affords the physician an opportunity to observe how the patient moves when he is not thinking that he is being directly observed. The caretaker should not be invited to the examination, so that the physician has a chance to talk to the patient alone. Very often an interesting contrast will be seen between the patient's responses with the caretaker present and the patient's responses when alone. Ask the patient again about his life-style and contrast the report with that obtained in the presence of the caretaker. It is also possible to ask at this time about the relationship between the patient and the caretaker. Not uncommonly, a different impression is obtained when the patient reports independently.

While accompanying the patient to the examining room the physician should introduce casual conversation. It is an interesting reflection of the patient's emotional involvement in his pain if he appears distressed and in great difficulty when he talks about his pain but can speak casually and conversationally about the weather, the latest football scores, or other topics that interest him. A marked discrepancy between the demeanor of the patient while describing his symptoms and while engaging in other conversation might also indicate that he is trying to oversell the physician on the seriousness of his complaint.

The physical examination begins with the initial observation of the patient. The patient who walked with the physician down the hall to the examining room with little difficulty may display considerable distress later when tested in the examining room. The patient who appeared comfortable and sociable while sitting in the waiting room may present a demeanor of profound distress as soon as the physician walks into the office.

The emotional tone of the patient is particularly important in evaluating chronic pain behavior. Note the patient's demeanor during the history. Is the patient agitated and distressed, or does he sit calmly and relate his story objectively? Does he speak in a monotone? Does he sit hunched forward in his chair, and furrow his brow in the picture of depression?

Observing the patient during walking is quite helpful. Having the patient walk on toes and heels may be revealing, particularly if he performs better with this difficult maneuver than with ordinary walking. Observation of the posture is important, not only from the standpoint of muscle symmetry and erect position of the trunk, but also as the posture denotes depression or other psychological problems which may bear on the chronic pain complaint.

A history of the patient's physical activities at home has already been taken. Does the mobility in the examining room correspond to that history? Does the patient who claims self care and relatively vigorous activity need help putting on his shoes? Does the patient who reports complete dependency undress and dress without difficulty?

One significant situation which is generally not described but usually represents important secondary gain is that of the patient who requires special consideration coming to the examination, particularly when the demonstrable physical disability does not justify the need for such special consideration. Thus, the patient who is relatively mobile by history and physical examination but requires an ambulance to come to the office may be setting the stage for an overevaluation of his problem. The patient who 'becomes ill' while sitting in the waiting room and requires special assistance to lie down in the examining room until the doctor arrives is suspect, unless sufficient physical cause for such behavior can be found. Usually, patients who exaggerate in such a manner are accompanied by excessively concerned spouses or caretakers who sit with them in the examining room holding their hands, wiping their brows, providing medication, and generally rewarding the pain behavior.

Inappropriate responses during the examination itself should be noted, just as discrepancies between examination and pre-examination behavior were noted. The patient who hyper-reacts when a cold stethoscope is placed on the chest – not a painful stimulus – may react the same way to minor discomfort, in which case there is a tendency to overtreat the patient. The patient who dramatically displays pain response on palpation of a muscle and then responds just as dramatically to compression of a fold of overlying skin between the fingers may be experiencing no muscle tenderness at all. On the other hand, deep palpation of muscles in spasm or palpable nodules in the muscle may give credence to the patient's report of tenderness. One must be suspicious of the patient who exhibits extreme distress on straight leg raising to 5 or 10° during the testing, if the examiner can elevate the straight leg 60–80° while distracting the patient during some other part of the examination. The claims of patients who are unable to bend more than 5° during the examination but are able to tie their own shoe laces with no difficulty are certainly suspect.

One curious sign is the patient who clutches a tissue during the interview. Those patients, usually female, have a very high incidence of functional overlay to the pain complaints.

An important part of the physical examination is *assessing the reliability of the findings,* particularly subjective findings. For instance, one must not only note the report of sensory impairment on testing, but also interpret whether the finding appears to be valid.

It is no longer appropriate to divide positive findings into 'functional' or 'organic'. There is a continuum between these points. A patient's perception will be colored to various degrees by the emotional factors discussed throughout this volume. Nor is it appropriate to consider that a positive finding without an explainable organic basis is either hysterical pain or malingering, since the examination can also be colored by such factors as depression, somatic preoccupation or conditioned responses.

Remember that the *sensory examination* is entirely subjective, and the motor examination is partly so. In the sensory examination, the physician must rely entirely on the patient's report and must interpret the accuracy of that report as well as the distribution of any sensory loss.

Areas of anesthesia are more frequently seen in hysteria than in malingering. However, the distribution of sensory loss may fail to correspond to the pattern of organic innervation. It is often said that stocking-like anesthesia is an indication of hysteria, but the physician must be aware that it may also occur in peripheral neuropathy. It is not uncommon for patients with bona fide herniated discs to have hypesthesia over the entire leg, although it may be more marked in the distribution of the involved nerve root.

If there is an area of sensory loss or decrease, make note of the border with a small ink mark. Later in the examination, come back and test the area again with the patient's eyes closed, and look for inconsistencies.

We have found a Wartenberg pinwheel to be far better for testing for sensory loss than repeated sticks with a needle. Not only does the pinwheel apply the stimulus with consistent intensity, but borders of sensory loss can be quite accurately defined by rolling the pinwheel from the less sensitive to more sensitive area. When testing the border of sensory loss to confirm a suspicion of an inorganic pattern, it is helpful to run the pinwheel directly across the line of demarcation one time, then diagonally and with varying curved patterns, to see if the border is at a consistent area of the skin or whether it changes depending on the track of the stimulus or the speed at which the pinwheel is moved.

If the change in sensation occurs abruptly at the midline, the physician should be suspicious, because ordinarily there is a small area of overlap. If the midline border for touch and pinstick sensation involves the head or the area over the sternum, the physician can then test on both sides of the midline of the forehead or sternum with a tuning fork. Because the entire bone or cartilage vibrates en masse, there should be no abrupt transition of vibratory sensation at the midline. If there is, the cause is not of organic nature.

The *motor examination* of the undraped patient begins with the general body build and muscle tone. Solid, well-defined muscles with no limitation of motion would not be likely in a patient who claims to have been strictly bedridden for the last 6 months. Calloused and grimy hands are inappropriate for a patient who claims he has done no physical labor for the last year. The body of a patient who claims to have been extremely inactive should look the part.

If weakness is found on examination which, from the nature of the injury, should be of lower motor neuron type, there should be accompanying atrophy and reflex changes. Weakness secondary to upper motor neuron disease may or may not be associated with hyperreflexia.

When paralysis is strictly the result of malingering, the patient may actively resist the physician's moving the extremity. When being tested for motor strength, the patient who is not performing to his maximum ability will often allow resistance of the part to be overcome in short, jerking movements, rather than by giving way gradually as in organic weakness. If this occurs, the patient may be told directly that he is not trying as hard as he could. A change in his performance following that admonition confirms the impression. Also, when the physician is able to partially extend the extremity against the patient's resistance, the extremity should suddenly pull back when the physician abruptly lets go. If the extremity remains in its partially flexed position, this may indicate that the patient was simultaneously contracting antagonists to make the extremity appear weaker.

On repeated grasping, the patient with organic weakness generally fatigues rapidly, whereas in simulated paralysis the patient may show an increase in strength rather than progressive fatigue.

The largest group of chronic pain patients falls somewhere in the middle of the continuum we described earlier. These may be patients with bona fide organic disease, or at least a history of such disease or injury. The exaggeration of the symptoms may be the result of an emotional need for suffering. The patient may have an exaggerated perception of the pain because of underlying bias in his perception, which may originate within or may be implanted by a family member, attorney, or physician.

It is virtually impossible to determine where a patient is on the continuum, that is, how much psychological contribution there is to the pain or how much of a patient's biased pain report is conscious and how much unconscious. Nevertheless, physicians are frequently called upon to pinpoint the degree of functional disability in compensation cases. Compensation carriers should recognize the emotional problems which can result from physical injury and the resultant disability. Unfortunately, the term which has come to represent such problems, 'post-traumatic neurosis,' does little more than pretend that psychological factors are easily classified.

For treatment purposes, the physician should recognize – and explain to the patient – that there is evidence of psychological contribution to the pain perception or report. The initial patient interview, in which the problem is defined, is the ideal time for this explanation. The patient's

motives should not be challenged; it should not be implied that he is malingering, that the pain is hysterical pain, or that it is 'all in your head'.
Any such implication could cause the patient to seek medical attention
elsewhere or redouble his efforts to justify disability. The statement, 'I can
find no evidence of organic disease,' should be followed by an invitation
to work together on all factors which are contributing to the patient's disability.

Some general comments apply to *examination of the pain complaint,*
regardless of the body part involved. The patient should be asked to demonstrate the specific *distribution* of the pain. Indeed, it is helpful to request
that same demonstration several times during the examination in order to
compare reports. The patient who has very specific pain of a finite etiology
will generally define the distribution of the pain exactly the same way each
time. A patient who is complaining more of distress than pain is likely to be
very inconsistent about the distribution of his pain. It is often more helpful
to have the patient outline the area of the pain on his body rather than
trying to infer from a description which may not convey the information
accurately.

Beware of the patient whose pain follows an extremely elaborate distribution. The pain that winds around, through, up, and back down an
extremity or overlaps trunk and extremities is very often not of organic
origin and may have been elaborated unduly by the patient.

After the patient has defined the area of pain, the next step is to observe
and explore the painful area for clues to the etiology. This simple part of the
examination is somehow often overlooked because it cannot be defined as a
specific 'test'. Nevertheless, it is perhaps the most important part of the
evaluation of the chronic pain complaint.

Note the *appearance* of the area of pain. Is there discoloration, ery-
thema or atrophy? Is there scarring? Is there dermatitis from the use of a
heating pad? Does the patient guard the area in a manner appropriate to his
complaints, or is the area guarded in an excessively dramatic fashion.

Palpate the area. Does it feel different from the surrounding area? Is
there nodularity or a firmness of the skin? Is it warmer than the surrounding
areas? On deep palpation, is there a feeling of fullness or asymmetry? Is
there palpable muscle spasm as the fingers are rolled back and forth across
the underlying muscle?

Search for tenderness. Ask the patient to report when palpation produces pain. Ask further that the patient report when *'the'* tender spot is
palpated.

Try to define in which tissue layer the pain originates. Begin by brushing the skin lightly. Is a light touch interpreted as pain? If so, does this represent causalgia, or is the patient's tolerance so low that any sensation is interpreted as pain?

Palpate the skin and subcutaneous layer. Does the patient report as much pain when the skin and subcutaneous fat are pinched between the fingers as when deep palpation is applied to the muscles? If so, one must question whether the musculoskeletal system actually is producing pain.

Then palpate firmly enough to press on the underlying muscle and fascia. Is the muscle body in symmetry with that on the other side? Is there palpable muscle spasm when the fingers are rubbed transversely across the muscle body? Is there a nodularity in the muscle which may represent old muscle tearing and resultant areas of fibrous tissue scarring?

Have the patient report if there is tenderness on palpation of the muscle. Is the tenderness sharply confined? Is it diffuse? If so, does it extend longitudinally along a single muscle bundle, which would represent a spasm of that muscle, or does it extend diffusely over several muscles, which might represent anything? If there is muscle tenderness, does it correspond to the area of the patient's chief complaint of pain? If there is muscle tenderness, what is the patient's response if you then go back to more superficial palpation?

If the area of tenderness involves part of the body that can be manipulated or moved, such as an extremity, does *manipulation* of that area correspond to the impression obtained on palpation of the muscle? If the area is reported to be tender on palpation, but the muscle can be stretched with no difficulty, one must question whether the report of tenderness is accurate. On the other hand, if the muscle cannot be stretched at all, but there is no tenderness whatsoever, one must consider the joint as well as the muscle as a possible etiology of the pain.

All of this is designed to identify the tissue that might be the origin of the pain. If the tissue plane can be identified, suggestions for treatment will naturally follow. It is useless to treat a pain of subcutaneous origin with a muscle conditioning program, and likewise, highly unlikely that extreme tenderness on skin and subcutaneous palpation would respond to trigger point or local anesthetic blocks in the muscle.

Many patients with chronic pain have pain of musculotendinous origin. They usually have been immobilized sufficiently to experience major deterioration of mobility so that they have pain on any motion. Consequently an examination of the musculoskeletal system is an important part of the chronic pain evaluation.

1. Myofascial Syndrome

Myofascial syndrome, for the purpose of this discussion, is defined as pain which follows local injury to an area of muscle or attachment of muscle to bone. The injury usually results from sudden forced stretching or tearing of muscle, particularly muscle held in contraction, such as in a rear-end collision or trying to lift too heavy a weight. The syndrome may also occur at the site of a surgical incision or where muscle has been incised or dissected from bone during surgery, for example, at a laminectomy site or a donor site for a fusion. There may be only pain and tenderness in the area or there may be associated muscle spasm. On examination, a trigger point may be revealed, that is, a localized area of muscle tenderness on deep palpation, very often associated with palpable muscle spasm as well. The local nature of the problem may be confirmed by the alleviation of pain on infiltration of the trigger point with local anesthetic. There may be referred pain radiating down the same dermatome, which may also disappear on infiltration of the trigger point.

The most common locations for chronic intractable musculoskeletal pain are the cervical and low back areas. There are many reasons, one being the poor design of the spine for the erect posture. Muscles of the back and neck are under constant tension in fulfilling their function to support the erect body. Spinal reflexes and tonic neck reflexes are always at play to maintain sufficient tension to adjust the posture and head position. Poor posture causes skeletal and ligamentous systems to work less efficiently in holding the spine erect, so the difference must be made up by increasing the muscle tension.

Since the trunk and neck muscles are always under tension as part of their supporting function, they are more vulnerable to tearing and injury on sudden flexion, extension or jolting. Also, since they are always under tension, it is not possible to put them completely at rest to allow healing once an injury has occurred. Lying in bed helps to decrease the tension of the back muscles significantly, far less so the cervical muscles. To make matters worse, muscles of the trunk reflexly increase their tension during times of emotional stress or tension. The resultant increased muscle tension may augment musculoskeletal pain originating from those muscles and certainly may prolong the pain by many weeks or even months. Since these same muscles increase tension on emotional tension, fatigue or depression, the vicious cycle is set up of pain, depression and tension, increased muscle contraction causing increased pain, and so forth.

There are several points to be noted about the examination of patients with musculoskeletal pain of the back or neck. Patients with musculoskeletal pain of the posterior cervical area may complain of pain in the neck, shoulders, or arms, or they may complain of headache. For any of those complaints, attention should be directed to the examination of the neck muscles. If the pain is manifest as headache, particularly headache which has the characteristics of tension headaches, the suboccipital or upper cervical muscles are frequently tender or painful. The patient should be asked to move the neck through full range of motion, including rotation, flexion, extension, and tilting (placing the ear on the ipsilateral shoulder). Extreme flexion or extension of the neck may intensify the patient's pain. There is frequently tenderness on palpation of the suboccipital area in the hollow just lateral to the long cervical muscles, just behind the lateral mass of the C_2 vertebra. In fact, pressing in this area may significantly provoke the patient's pain or headache, and infiltration of this area with local anesthetic (care being taken not to inject into the vertebral artery or spinal canal) may result in dramatic relief of the pain.

2. Low Back Pain

The examination for low back pain as it is ordinarily described is an excellent examination for the detection of a herniated lumbar disc. However, only a small minority of patients with low back pain have disc herniation. We refer the reader to the more classical neurosurgical and orthopedic texts for an outline of the diagnostic examination for herniated disc.

There are several unique considerations in examining the low back of the patient with chronic pain of myofascial origin. As in herniated disc disease, the patient's posture is important. The patient usually does not assume the classical posture described for herniated disc, slightly bent over at the waist with one knee bent, weight supported on the other leg, and a list to one side. Instead, a patient with chronic low back pain may show only typical poor posture with a lordosis and sagging abdomen. Ability to bend at the waist may be limited, particularly in a patient who has been inactive for some time. On straight leg raising, this limited ability from disused muscles may be manifest as posterior thigh or low back pain at 45–60° because of tight hamstring muscles, in contrast to pain of radicular distribution caused by disc herniation. To differentiate between tight hamstrings and radicular pain, the patient should be asked precisely where the pain is. Palpation of the hamstring group when under stretch may make the pain worse; that is, stretching the tight hamstring muscle may make it more subject to tenderness on palpation. Very often, the muscles of both legs are symmetrically impaired, but the pain may be referred to one side of the back if there is a unilateral lumbar muscle strain. Bending is often done poorly, with the hands going to the knees or slightly below. Attempts at further bending are restricted mechanically, or by patient complaint of back or posterior upper leg pain.

With unilateral lumbar muscle strain, the patient may have a list to one side, which can be differentiated from a scoliosis. If an imaginary plumb line is dropped from the spinous process of C_7 it falls at the crease of the buttocks in scoliosis because of the compensatory curve. However, if the patient has a list, it falls off to one side. On X-ray, scoliosis has a rotatory component, whereas a list is tilting without rotation of the vertebrae.

When a patient has a list because of lumbar muscle strain, the list will be toward the side of the pain, whereas with a herniated disc it may be to either side. The muscle group may be particularly tender when palpated with the patient standing. When the patient is lying prone, palpable muscle spasm may be apparent, and this may coincide with local muscle tenderness. A word of caution, however – a patient with a herniated disc may have unilateral lumbar muscle spasm as well. In order to differentiate, look for other signs of radiculopathy.

3. Trigger Points

A frequently encountered concomitant of lumbar muscle strain or a myofascial syndrome is the occurrence of trigger points. These are small areas of the muscle that are tender to very deep palpation. The tenderness is usually sharply localized and may be associated with a nodular feeling of the muscle in that area. Such trigger points may represent areas in which the muscle was torn during an injury. They may represent nodular fibrosis or localized spasm, and may potentiate local pain and muscle spasm for many months. For some reason, they are not extensively described in most literature concerning low back problems.

The search for trigger points can be a particularly helpful maneuver in evaluating patients with chronic intractable back pain. The patient lies prone and the examiner presses firmly about the general area of pain searching for specific points which are tender or painful on very deep palpation. Often pressure on such trigger points will reproduce the patient's presenting symptom of pain or may even cause referred pain which travels down the leg in a seemingly radicular distribution. Sometimes the trigger points are identified only by pain on deep palpation. Other times, muscle spasm or local nodularity will verify the diagnosis.

The most common sites in the low back for trigger points are just above the posterior iliac spine, the crest of the sacrum, the upper end of the sacroiliac joint (where the long muscles of the back attach to the upper margin of the sacrum and adjacent ileum), just lateral to a laminectomy or fusion incision, at the iliac crest, over the sacral foramina, or over the donor site after a fusion has been performed.

To document the trigger points, they are marked in ink on palpation of the back. A 1½ inch hypodermic needle is inserted at the mark designating each trigger point and is advanced until the patient's report of sudden severe pain indicates that the tip of the needle has entered the trigger area. This is most often just at the depth of the bone or the muscular attachment to the bone, or may occur as the examiner feels the needle penetrate the lumbodorsal fascia or ligamentum nuchae. 2–5 ml of local anesthetic may be injected at each area. Dramatic alleviation of the patient's pain provides evidence that the pain originates in the muscle or fascia of the lower back, rather than at a nerve root.

Results of diagnostic block with local anesthetic must be accepted with extreme caution, however, since they may be associated with considerable placebo effect. The patient who is enthusiastically hopeful of pain relief may receive a surprising degree of temporary benefit from an injection of any kind. Important to diagnosis is not only whether the patient has immediate relief on administration of the local anesthetic, but whether the pain returns after the local anesthetic wears off. Returning pain may even be somewhat worse due to the trauma of the injection. Pain relief may outlast the duration of anesthetic in some patients with myofascial syndrome. However, the patient who has too much relief from a local anesthetic block is just as worrisome as the patient who has insufficient relief.

A minimum of three or, ideally, four blocks should be done before one can conclude any benefit. At least one of the blocks should be with saline, and the patient's response to that block should be discernably different from the response to a local anesthetic block. The onset of pain relief should be prompt after injection of anesthetic and should be reflected by objective signs such as increased range of motion, as well as by subjective report. The pain should return about the time it is anticipated that the local anesthetic might wear off, and, as mentioned, it may even be worse for a time after that. For best evaluation, it is helpful to use lidocaine for the initial one or two blocks, followed by a saline injection, and then a bupivicaine block. Pain relief should be quite prompt after the lipocaine blocks, and perhaps delayed for a few minutes after the bupivicaine block. Relief after the lidocaine block might last for two to four hours, and four to eight hours after the bupivicaine block. Relief after the saline injection should be incomplete and transient, if it occurs at all. If the unprompted response follows this pattern, you can be reasonably assured that you have identified the tissue from which the pain originates.

Suggested Reading

1   DeJong, R.N.: The neurological examination; 4th ed. (Harper & Row, New York 1979).
2   Keim, H.A.: Low back pain. Clinical Symposia 25(3): 2–32 (1973).
3   Sternbach, R.A.: Pain patients, traits and treatment (Academic Press, New York 1974).
4   Travell, J.G.; Simons, D.G.: Myofascial pain and dysfunction: the trigger point manual (Williams & Wilkins, Baltimore 1983).

Chapter IX

Management

There are five aspects to a chronic pain management program: (A) re-definition of the problem, including management of psychosocial issues, (B) discontinuation of addicting medication, (C) techniques for control of pain perception, (D) remobilization, and, only after the above are well underway, (E) specific therapy, if appropriate.

Note that the treatment of the pain symptom per se is deferred and usually receives relatively low priority, because there is generally no adequate symptomatic treatment. By definition, if such treatment had existed, the patient never would have developed the chronic pain in the first place. At any rate, those symptomatic treatments that are available have a much lower success rate when used outside the context of a comprehensive chronic pain program. Indeed, the success rate with isolated symptomatic modalities is not much greater than could be expected from the placebo effect, but 80% of patients may benefit from a comprehensive program.

A. Redefinition of the Problem

The initial step in management of any patient with chronic pain is for both the patient and the physician to accept the chronic nature of the problem. It must be recognized and accepted that jumping from one ineffective treatment to another or one physician to another has been and will continue to be futile. Those treatments in particular should be abandoned which are appropriate for acute, but not for chronic, pain. A frank discussion should establish the fact that there is not a medical treatment for every pain, especially not for every chronic pain. This discussion-negotiation should set realistic, obtainable goals and attempt to insure that emotional resources will not be diverted from those goals. Thereafter the patient must assume responsibility for doing things himself, with the physician serving as guide. He is no longer allowed to be passive or to expect the doctor to take care of him.

We have emphasized that a major impediment to satisfactory management of chronic pain patients is their successful simulation of acute illness. The simulation, perfected through long-term assumption of the acute sick role, often persuades concerned physicians to attempt inappropriate interventions. Inevitably, the drugs, medical interventions, and surgeries add up to histories of treatment failures. At the same time, long-term sick role occupancy produces very real problems of its own which must be recognized and managed – such problems as disability, regression and illness insistence. These conditions are sanctioned and reinforced by the physician who continues to offer treatments aimed at the pain symptom as though the problem were an acute one. Almost none of the 600 consecutive patients reviewed in our pain service had treatable cause for the pain complaint, while all had long histories of unsuccessful treatment attempts. We consider this impressive evidence both of the power of illness insistence to elicit treatment responses and of the medical risks inherent in simulation of acute illness.

When thorough history and physical examination support the diagnosis of the chronic pain syndrome, conscientious physicians will alter their habitual mode of interaction with patients in two very important ways. First they will reject the patients' claims of acute illness, and second they will temporarily relinquish their roles as acute healers. Setting aside this role, one acquired through inclination, training, and practice, is difficult for most physicians. Likelihood that chronic pain patients will encounter physicians who can suspend their acute treatment orientation is further decreased by the number of times these patients are referred to other physicians for acute interventions. As referrals to ever more specialized physicians multiply, so do chances that the new physician will be one who is more comfortable with sophisticated diagnostic and treatment procedures than with rehabilitative management. The generalists who continually refer these patients and repeatedly attempt to rule out medical illness are also contributing to the patient's belief that an undiagnosed illness is present.

When treatments fail, the physician's frustrations and realization that the problem was misrepresented and misinterpreted lead to 'back end' efforts to convince the patient that 'there is nothing more to be done'. Such statements are often accompanied by suggestions for further referral or psychiatric consultation, the latter with its implication that 'the problem is all in your head'. The referral along with the physician's undisguisable frustration are interpreted by patients as rejection and a threat to continued sanction of their sick role occupancy. Patient and physician are disappointed, if not outrightly angry.

If the physician can step outside the role of acute healer, this pattern can be broken and the first constructive steps toward management taken. Constructive management begins with a redefinition of the problem as a chronic one and restatement of the goal as rehabilitation. Patients who accept the new diagnosis and goal are candidates for rehabilitation. They are re-evaluated in light of the newly defined problem, using their histories and routine examination and diagnostic techniques. Careful history should solicit details of the patient's premorbid social functioning which can serve as useful guides in setting realistic goals for rehabilitation. Management interventions then naturally follow, aimed initially at reversing disability and regression, products of acute illness simulation.

We have suggested that chronic pain patients can be divided into four identifiable groups (table I, Chapter V). The major portion of this chapter applies to psychosocial management of all chronic pain patients. Two groups – those with psychogenic pain and those whose personality indicates a need to suffer – are given special attention at the end of the chapter.

A psychiatric counseling program serves a multitude of purposes. It is part of the program for the treatment of depression and resocialization. Its concerns are the setting and attaining of realistic goals. It combats regression and hopelessness. It addresses the role played by secondary gain in the perpetuation of regression and disability. It redefines the role of caretaker as one of support for rehabilitation efforts.

Every comprehensive program for the treatment of chronic pain has a psychiatric component. Some may be behaviorally oriented, others more analytical in nature. Some may involve an almost religious ritual, others may be very loosely structured. It is becoming recognized that the specific nature of the psychiatric program does not appear to influence the success rate. The common denominator is that the counseling aspect of the program educates the patient about the unique nature of chronic pain and provides the moral support and encouragement he needs throughout the program.

The psychiatric program in a comprehensive chronic pain management plan is unlike the typical psychiatric consultation obtained in isolation from a chronic pain program. The latter will often conclude, 'The patient is depressed. Of course the patient is depressed; he has had pain for the last 6 months. Treat his pain and then send him back to me pain-free and I will take care of his depression.' Obviously useless advice!

Psychiatric intervention for treatment of pain is appropriate for the few patients with primary psychogenic pain whose management is discussed elsewhere. The majority of pain patients either resist a referral to a psychiatrist, viewing such a referral as denial of their illness, or go grudgingly to convince the referring physician that his pain is real. We think that counseling can be effective in helping patients face and resolve the problems in living that are inextricably tied to their pain symptoms. It is most important, however, that patients realize they are not seeking counseling as a treatment for the pain. Addressing the psychiatric management as part of a comprehensive program allows the patient to accept psychiatric care without feeling defensive, which is a major function of a chronic pain clinic.

It is only after the patient accepts the redefinition of his problem as chronic pain, rather than acute pain, that a treatment program can be considered. As long as the patient goes from doctor to doctor trying medication after medication and treatment after treatment, he is unable to use his resources to find an acceptable life-style compatible with his physical problem. Lying back and waiting for a 'magical cure' is the hallmark of the regressed and dependent state. Although the patient may always hold some hope that future developments will provide physical help, he must choose between waiting incapacitated and in pain until such future developments occur or working to develop his potential to the fullest.

By far the majority of chronic pain syndrome patients seek sick role status as a means of escaping unpleasant responsibilities or overwhelming problems. They credit their pain with being the single cause for their inability to function as responsible adults. A primary management objective, therefore, is enabling the patient to understand how he is misusing his pain. A systematic exploration of the patient's real conflicts – financial, personal, marital or work-related – is undertaken to break up what has been seen as one overwhelming problem into smaller concerns that can be investigated and resolved. Patients learn that their pain is not the underlying problem they claim it is, but is a symptom of stress or conflict. Pain should come to be interpreted as a signal to 'do something' about a real problem rather than an excuse for not addressing problems.

In the process, patients become educated about pain. They should learn, for example, that (1) most chronic pain is not an indication of physiological damage, (2) stress, depression, fatigue and poor general health lower tolerance to pain regardless of its origin, and (3) the perception of pain is a psychological event and is subject to control and modification by cognitive techniques. Natural childbirth (the Lamaze method) illustrates this last point. In natural childbirth, an understanding of what is happening together with employment of pain control techniques can successfully reduce pain perception.

We have found that redefining the problem for the patient is actually a four-step process.

First, the patient is confronted with our clinical judgment that there is no mechanical or illness process present that will respond to definitive treatment.

Second, and more important, the patient's extensive medical history, characterized by lack of response to acute drugs and surgeries, is reviewed as further testimony to the chronic nature of the current pain.

This leads to the *third* step, which is explaining to the patient the differences between acute and chronic pain and the ways in which each is treated, for example (although you will tailor your terminology to the patient's background), 'Someone with an acute injury or acute pain expects the doctor to diagnose the problem and institute a treatment that will lead to cure and return to normal function. This is certainly what we all hope for and, obviously, what you still expect. Unfortunately, your pain is not that kind of problem. Chronic pain, like any chronic problem, cannot be cured. Its management requires an approach markedly different from approaches to acute problems.'

'In chronic pain, what is wrong is not as important as controlling pain perception and the subsequent disability and regression. Inactivity, being able to do fewer things for yourself, and waiting for a doctor to treat your pain cause regression and inability to function socially as before. These conditions are experienced in acute illness also, but are temporary. In your case, the pain, disability, and regression are elements in a self-perpetuating process. Ironically this is often aggravated by the kind of pain medications and tranquilizers you have been taking. While these can be useful for temporary relief of acute pain, they not only do not relieve chronic pain, but actually cause additional problems such as depression, drug dependence, and further decrease in ability to function socially.'

In the *fourth* and final step we outline the choices the patient has, as follows: 'For these reasons, we feel that you have an important decision to make. You may choose to continue your search for a physician who can cure your pain, or you can accept that there is no cure for your chronic pain and decide to work toward managing it. The former choice is the response expected from those with acute injuries or illnesses, but is one we feel unlikely to be rewarding, given your history and our recent evaluation of your problem. If you can accept that you will not be exactly the way you were before all this began, that your main problems now are disability and regression, and that your chief goals are management of pain perception and minimization of disability, we can recommend a program and work with you so that you might develop better ways to cope with your chronic pain.'

This general statement is modified for such individual patient circumstances as evidence of drug addiction, significant clinical depression or issues related to compensation or lawsuits. If it is apparent that compensation is regarded by the patient as desirable and dependent upon continued disability or that a lawsuit is thought to promise substantial financial reward, we confront the matter directly. Where compensation is at stake, we express willingness to work with the patient toward the goal of replacing compensation benefits with gains from some type of work. If, however, it is clear that the patient is not going to get well until a lawsuit is settled, we suggest return to the clinic after that time.

The redefinition, with its rejection of the patient's claim to acute illness, is accompanied by sympathy and understanding of their hope for cure. Nonetheless, the point that all evidence accords with a diagnosis of chronic pain is firmly made. The goal of rehabilitation and the physician's readiness to work with the patient toward achieving it are established during the initial doctor-patient contact. The advantages are obvious of such an approach over back-end attempts to imply that nothing is wrong (when much is) or that the pain is in the patient's head.

In our experience, patient responses to the redefinition fall roughly into three categories. The vast majority express disappointment but, in the end, are receptive to the new approach. Central to gaining their acceptance is the physician's ability to listen to their disappointment, to sympathize with their desire that things were different, and to work with them on the new program. There are two alternative responses. A surprising few, saying, in effect, 'I was afraid you were going to say that,' accept the redefinition and return to work without further treatment. An equally interesting response is voiced by members of another minority who reject the redefinition with the statement, 'I'm going back to my other doctor. He thinks I'm sick.' Both responses testify to our contention that physician sanction of sick role occupancy contributes materially to perpetuation of chronic pain syndrome. We tell those who wish to return to a previous physician or continue to search for a cure (about 5% of our clinic patients) that we doubt they will find a doctor with a magical cure, but that we understand their need to pursue the possibility and will be happy to work with them if they change their minds. With those who accept our redefinition and goals, we embark on the next step, negotiation of a management program.

1. Negotiation of a Management Program

Negotiations for rehabilitation are best undertaken with the patient and spouse or other family members. Family cooperation in rehabilitation efforts is critical to success of the program. Family members must learn not to reinforce pain behaviors and not to foster regression and disability by 'nursing' the patient. Spouses, in their adaptation to the chronic illness, often present special problems. In one typical pattern of response, spouses become frustrated and resentful of the sacrifices they must make, then guilty over their feelings of resentment. Other spouses resolve the situation by assuming a comfortable caretaker role. We have found that women sometimes cling to the patient role for gratification of dependency needs and in fear that if they did not need caring for, their husbands might leave them. Men, for their part, may cling to patienthood for gratification of similar dependency needs which their notion of the masculine role would not allow them to claim if they were not sick. Illness, then, preserves mothering and conceals the need to deal with serious personal and marital problems.

2. Establishing Realistic Goals

Redefining the goal for the family as well as for the patient generally forces discussion of obvious problems that are not illness-related. This initiates the necessary process of understanding how sick role occupancy has been used to excuse personal and interpersonal conflicts which the patient has avoided facing with the explanation, 'If it were not for this pain I would be able to ...' Negotiation can be considered accomplished when patients and their families understand the readjustment that rehabilitation will demand from all of them and agree to cooperate on all aspects of the management regimen.

The dual intention of the psychosocial interventions is recognition of patient responsibility for pain management and replacement of illness insistence with well behavior. To achieve this goal, psychosocial management interventions must address as many psychological contributors to the patient's disabling problem as possible. These include depression, regression, physician manipulation, illness insistence and, in a few instances, psychogenic pain or a personality that indicates a need to suffer.

3. Treatment of Depression

It is normal to be depressed after months of pain and/or disability. The depression in itself causes a vicious cycle with a deterioration of pain tolerance, further regression, and hopelessness which interferes with any rehabilitation effort, which increases the depression, and so forth. All of the aspects of the chronic pain program combine to combat depression. However, some parts of the program direct themselves more specifically to depression: (a) withdrawal of pain medication, (b) withdrawal of tranquilizers, (c) institution of antidepressant medications, (d) establishment of realistic goals, (e) psychiatric counseling, (f) resocialization and reversal of regression.

It is unlikely that any program intended to treat depression can be successful unless pain medications are discontinued. Not only are antidepressant medications very helpful in the management of chronic depression, but there is some evidence that some of them, particularly the tricyclic antidepressants, may have a specific analgesic effect for chronic pain, which makes them the only medication with such an effect. Thus, antidepressants constitute the foundation for the pharmacological aspects of any chronic pain program.

The prolonged disability inherent in sick role occupancy that is responsible for regression also leads to secondary depression. A survey of 200 consecutive pain patients using various objective scales of depression found the average chronic pain patient to be only slightly depressed, but clinical depression is a major contributor to disability in a small group of patients. Tricyclic antidepressants are most effective in this group and, in fact, we have found them helpful in treating most chronic pain patients. Both depression and regression lower pain threshold physiologically and lead to psychological states in which one is more preoccupied with bodily perceptions. Tricyclics appear to raise pain threshold independent of their antidepressant effect and seem also to help in drawing patients out of their regressed state.

4. Treatment of Regression

With redefinition of the problem as a chronic one, the sanction for acute sick behavior is revoked. Thus, redefinition is perhaps the most pivotal step in reversing regression. If the patient does not acknowledge, rationally and emotionally, that the problem is a chronic one and cannot be cured, other attempts at reversing regression are doomed.

The key to overcoming regression can be simply stated: The patient must become more independent and able to care for himself. Physician and family or caretakers must be adamant in refusing to accept responsibility for the chronic condition. The first step may vary from insisting that the patient get up from bed daily, come to the table for meals, dress himself, engage in exercise, or resume some household or work obligation – this depends upon the degree of regression.

The primary medical intervention discussed later on – withdrawal of narcotic analgesics, barbiturates, and simple tranquilizers – goes far toward increasing the patient's independence and ability to interact socially and thus toward reversing regression. Treatment with tricyclic antidepressants, if indicated for depression and if successful in trial, may also help the patient to regain his premorbid, less dependent state.

The salutary effects that remobilization and pain control techniques can have on reversing regression just barely take second place to the primary goals of these procedures. Patient satisfaction with being able to resume some activity, on the one hand, and with being able to take some control over pain, on the other, goes far toward increasing a sense of independence and an unwillingness to gain attention through the repertoire of regressed behaviors previously relied upon.

5. The Manipulative Patient

Much has been written about the manipulative behavior of chronic pain patients. A particularly good book to which the reader is directed is *R.A. Sternbach's* 'Games Pain Patients Play'. From a management standpoint, the primary issue is the patient's presentation as an acutely ill person who requires active treatment by a doctor when the situation is, in reality, neither acute nor urgent. We have stressed how important it is for the doctor to recognize this primary manipulation of the doctor-patient relationship and to redefine the problem as chronic.

Permitting patients to become more childlike also encourages demanding and manipulative behavior. Here patients attempt to maneuver the physician into caring for them and accepting the responsibility for their illness.

There are two goals or aspects to the manipulation. First, patients wish to be sanctioned as acutely ill and relieved of responsibility. A second goal of manipulative behavior is recreation of the relationship between child and parent that the patient had experienced in the past. Histories can be helpful here, particularly inquiries into experiences patients have had with other illness and other physicians. A great deal of the patient's effort is directed toward engaging and keeping the physician very actively involved in the relationship rather than with rehabilitation – the real project at hand.

In response, physicians must remain firm, make clear what they have to offer – guidance and direction – and insist upon the patient's assuming responsibility for management of the chronic problem. A striking example of a group of manipulative patients is the 'need-to-suffer' group. At the conclusion to this chapter, we will offer some suggested goals and strategies for use with the need-to-suffer patient.

6. Behavior Modification

Because an etiology cannot be identified for the pain these patients experience and only rarely can the pain be obliterated, much of the management is directed toward changing the patient's behavior so that 'pain' does not mean 'sick' or 'disabled'. One way in which behavior change can be conceptualized and understood is by considering the learning theory rather than the medical or disease model of illness.

Learning theory recognizes that behavior is more than a mere response or outward expression of one's personality structure and development. Behavior is also an *operant,* itself capable of producing a result or reaction in the environment. When a given behavior is found to produce certain consequences, it is thereafter chosen or avoided in an attempt to control the immediate environment. If the chosen behavior elicits the desired response, it is reinforced and likely to occur with greater intensity, frequency, or both. If an agreeable reaction does not follow, the behavior is likely to diminish in intensity or frequency or perhaps disappear altogether. This model is particularly applicable to chronic pain behavior.

You have undoubtedly observed many examples of such operant behavior, which can be summarized in many cases as 'the squeaky wheel gets the grease'. Patients who exhibit a vocal and dramatic display of distress are more likely to be rewarded by being able to avoid work and responsibility, being allowed to regress, being taken care of by a spouse or relative (who otherwise might be disinterested and independent), and being allowed to get high on medications sanctified by a physician's prescription. As such behavior occurs time after time and the rewards are obtained repeatedly, the behavior becomes more and more ingrained. What has happened is that conditioning has occurred to promote the behavior that is being rewarded.

After such a conditioning process has occurred for some time, as is inevitable in chronic pain patients, pain behavior becomes reinforced to the point at which it is the natural behavior of the pain patient. In order to reverse that behavior, one must reverse the conditioning process through deconditioning.

'Well behavior' should be rewarded by encouragement, gratification, attention, and recognition. 'Sick behavior' should be punished by nonresponse, that is, by ignoring the patient when he complains of pain. Specifically, the taking of medication, reporting of pain, resting from activity, dependency, lack of social responsiveness, and avoidance of tasks should not be reinforced while their opposites should be.

Formal behavioral modification programs are advised if there is reason to suspect that reinforcement of well behavior would not proceed on its own. In such instances, admission to inpatient comprehensive pain units should be considered, as it should if the referring physician is inexperienced in directing rehabilitation or if the patient resists any aspect of the management program.

Group meetings of patients with similar problems can be invaluable to success. Patients who have progressed toward rehabilitation serve as models and sources of support for those who are beginning. They can also be very effective 'confronters' when patients regress or slip into any one of the 'pain games' so familiar to all in the group.

To be effective, operant conditioning must take place in a controlled environment, usually an inpatient chronic pain or psychosomatic unit, where staff members understand and cooperate with all aspects of the program. The greatest obstacle to successful substitution of well behavior is the complicity of the patient's family in the maintenance of patienthood. *Fordyce,* a proponent and initiator of operant conditioning for chronic pain management, found no significant decrease in pain intensity or associated disability reported by patients after their dismissal from the controlled setting, despite the fact that the family and caretakers had been educated to the objectives of the program.

It must be made clear, as *Fordyce* emphasizes, that operant conditioning is neither psychotherapy nor pain relief. It focuses on behavior-consequence relationships, not on conflict resolution or personality change. Likewise, the question is moot as to whether pain, defined independently of the pain behaviors, is changed. The purpose of operant conditioning is to depose pain as a primary force in social interaction while allowing other aspects of the management program to address psychological and pain issues if necessary.Thus, the role of operant conditioning is not to decrease the pain itself, but to treat the resultant disability. As has been discussed, the presence of disability and its attendant depression adversely affect the pain patient and, indeed, enhance the perception of pain. The goal is to lessen the disability by depriving the patient of the benefits of such disability, in anticipation that minimizing disability will lead to lessening of pain.

7. Psychogenic Pain

Two small groups of chronic pain patients were given separate profiles and special management consideration in Chapter V, patients with psychogenic pain and those with a personality structure that indicates a need to suffer. Inasmuch as their management differs somewhat from the general management plan we have just discussed, we will summarize specific interventions for these two groups here.

Patients with psychogenic pain, as you recall, have pain symptoms secondary to psychopathology, and we classified five types. Their pain may be a symptom of depression, a delusional symptom of psychosis, a symptom of anxiety, a conversion symptom of hysterical neurosis or a symptom of unresolved grief. It may help to review the case examples of these five types of psychogenic pain before looking at the suggested interventions which follow.

When clinical *depression* is the primary cause of pain, the pain typically disappears when the depression is treated. In most cases, clinical depression responds to a 3-week trial treatment with tricyclic antidepressants administered in the 100- to 200-mg/day range. Response indicates that treatment should be continued for about 2 months. It makes little difference which tricyclic antidepressant is used so long as adequate doses are taken over a long enough period of time. Physician familiarity with the drug and observation of the patient are important in light of the possible anti-cholinergic side-effects.

Psychiatric consultation is advised if the patient fails to respond to tricyclic antidepressants, if the physician is inexperienced in treating clinical depression, or if there is an exogenous situation which the patient needs help in handling. Electroconvulsive therapy has been used effectively in some depressions refractory to antidepressant therapy.

Where pain is a symptom of *delusional psychosis,* appropriate antipsychotic treatment or treatment of the underlying condition (e.g., toxic delirium) usually leads to disappearance of the delusional pain and other symptoms of psychosis.

Remember that with pain secondary to *anxiety* (as with that secondary to depression) differential diagnosis is based upon establishing that the anxiety (or depression) preceded onset of the pain complaint. As in the example case history, a situation that precipitates anxiety can usually be identified. When pain is secondary to anxiety, a two-step approach to management is taken. For example, in the most common type of pain secondary to anxiety – chest pain resulting from hyperventilation – the physiological chain of events responsible for the pain should be explained to the patient. After explaining the response mechanism, and, perhaps, having the patient demonstrate by overbreathing, the physician goes on to instruct the patient in how to manage the hyperventilation episode. Usually, engaging in brisk activity will help regulate the breathing. The most satisfactory intervention is to interrupt the chain of events before hyperventilaton begins. Often patients can do this by relaxing completely or holding their breath momentarily.

Successful management of patients with *conversion pain* as a *symptom of hysterical neurosis* can be difficult. The physician should reassure the patient that there is no evidence of serious medical illness or pathology, and should express confidence that the symptom will be short-lived. Those who fail to respond to reassurance and suggestion should be confronted with the lack of evidence of organic illness. The patient can be told that, in all likelihood, the pain is a manifestation of emotional stress and that return to activity will not be harmful. This information is frequently accepted with perplexity and anger. If, however, the physician demonstrates genuine concern and a willingness to help, these patients will very often agree to counseling or some form of social or psychiatric intervention.

When *unresolved grief* is recognized as underlying the pain complaint, initiation of grieving is the obvious management goal. Once initiated (or reinitiated) the grieving process will usually proceed as long as supportive listening continues. Those whose pain is grief-related are expected to feel worse before they feel better because they have been avoiding, through facsimile illness, the painful experience of grieving.

In general, where pain has a primary psychogenic cause, treatment of the pain as a symptom has no part in management. It is recognized that no medicine or surgery will relieve pain of psychologic origin. The underlying problem must be identified, accepted by the patient, and treated. In this respect, this group is more treatable than the balance of chronic pain patients. Their pain per se cannot be treated but there is, in each instance, an identifiable cause for the pain which can. Treatment ranges from antidepressant or antipsychotic medication to social service or psychiatric counseling. Critical to successful management is the treating physician's willingness to continue to see the patient even if referrals for other types of services are necessary.

Management of the patient whose personality indicates a *need to suffer* is especially challenging. Physicians, whose training and professional focus on the relieving of suffering have difficulty accepting that suffering is a necessary part of the way these people function. The theoretical management goal is to see that these patients suffer in their own best interest. On a practical level, this means protecting them from the consequences of unnecessary medical procedures, surgery, and iatrogenic drug dependence.

Like all chronic pain patients, members of this group should be made to understand that there is no definitive treatment for the kind of pain they have. Pain medications, as they already know, are ineffective. The burden of discontinuing drugs, remobilization, and reacceptance of social and family responsibilities should be substituted for the burden of pain.

We cannot overemphasize the importance of the physician's continued following of these patients. If they are seen at regularly scheduled times, even when they are doing well, their belief that suffering is the only means of attracting the attention of an important other person will not be reinforced.

B. Medications

Most chronic pain patients experience symptoms of depression secondary to their chronic pain and disability. Almost all medications which are used for treatment of acute pain add to the depression when given on a long-term basis. Particularly detrimental are narcotics and depressant tranquilizers.

Most chronic pain patients take many drugs, including narcotics, analgesics, minor tranquilizers, sedatives, major tranquilizers and possibly antidepressants, all for symptomatic relief. At the same time, their histories document and their personal testimony confirms that these drugs do not offer significant relief from pain. Many patients admit to taking them only to comply with doctors' orders or from a need to feel they are doing something about the pain. Further, prescription of drugs symbolizes to patients the doctor's belief that they have an illness which requires treatment.

As a group, these drugs reduce the patient's ability to function socially and thereby foster regression. In addition, each type of drug has its deleterious effects. The minor tranquilizers and sedatives are depressants which, with long-term use, lower pain tolerance and tend to induce both clinical depression and physical dependence. Narcotics are unsuitable for treatment of chronic pain, inasmuch as their continued use leads to tolerance and physical addiction with recurrent withdrawal. Major tranquilizers have been touted for use in chronic pain, but they carry the risk of serious neurological complications along with a tendency to reduce general social function. Antidepressants will be discussed in the next section.

1. Withdrawal of Medications
a) Analgesics

Most chronic pain patients are taking or have taken numerous inappropriate medications which have failed to alleviate their problem. Many also take excessive medication for physical problems which may have been misdiagnosed along the way in attempts to define an etiology for their pain. Pain patients tend to be medication oriented and may seek medications from more than one physician. There are only a few medications which are helpful in the treatment of chronic pain and its attendant depression. Consequently, the discussion of medical management will focus on discontinuation of inappropriate medication while defining the role of appropriate medication, particularly antidepressants, in chronic pain management.

No analgesics work for chronic pain. Because there is no satisfactory experimental model for chronic pain, those drugs which are tested pharmacologically and found to have analgesic properties are invariably tested in an experimental model of acute pain. Most affect the pain perception pathway or its transmitters somewhere along its course from periphery to the higher centers of the brain. The complaint of chronic pain, however, may be related primarily to distress and suffering, and the pain pathways may be only minimally involved. Indeed, after several months of chronic pain, a major component of the problem is not the pain per se but the resulting distress and disability.

No pain medication, with the exception of aspirin or similar drugs, can be used over a prolonged period of time without producing tolerance. This means that most analgesic medication must be taken in larger and larger doses in order to have any analgesic effect. Because of tolerance, the analgesic effects of a given dose, or even doses elevated to maximum safety limits, diminish with time, while unwanted side effects may persist or grow. For that reason, analgesic medications do not work for pain which persists more than a few weeks. This problem is only too well recognized by those who treat patients with cancer pain.

All analgesics, with the exception of several aspirin-like compounds, are varieties of narcotics. They possess the ability of narcotics to produce tolerance, habituation, and addiction, and, consequently, are not only inappropriate for long-term use, but are dangerous when given over a period of time.

Remember that each time you prescribe an analgesic medication, you are giving an addicting narcotic.

No narcotic should be prescribed under any circumstance without a definite plan for its discontinuation. When narcotics are prescribed postoperatively or after an injury, the physician can be reasonably certain that the acute pain will subside within several days and the narcotic discontinued. When a narcotic is given to a patient with cancer, the plan may be to continue it until the death of the patient, which may be imminent. If you prescribe a narcotic for a patient with chronic pain, when do you plan to discontinue it?

In all patients who have had pain relief after admission to the Chronic Pain Unit, the most significant step toward that relief was the withdrawal of narcotics. It is often recognized that the patient's most disabling symptoms were produced by the medication rather than the initiating physical problem. The patients are told prior to admission to the Chronic Pain Unit that they will receive no pain medication, and why. It is pointed out that if medication were the answer, they would be taking medication and not being admitted to the Chronic Pain Unit, so the very fact that they present themselves for treatment indicates that the medication has failed. It is emphasized that under no circumstances will they receive narcotics, regardless of what happens to their pain. They are warned that their pain will be worse during the period of withdrawal. They are also told that the discomfort of withdrawal will taper off in about 3 days, and that by 5–7 days they should feel much better. They are warned that their sleep pattern might be upset, and that it may take some time before they re-establish normal regulation of sleep.

Most patients who have demonstrated the pattern of recurrent narcotic withdrawal have significant relief from pain by the end of the first week, due mainly to the discontinuation of narcotics. Indeed, the effect is often so dramatic that decisions for specific treatments are deferred until the end of the first week, since very often a much less elaborate physical program is necessary than was originally considered.

In addition to the significant effect on addiction, the discontinuation of all narcotics has a markedly beneficial effect on the depression that most of the patients show. Narcotics are depressant. During the period of withdrawal, the depression is replaced by anxiety and agitation. As the withdrawal period ends, the effect of the narcotic on the patient's mood is also alleviated, and a more normal mood holds forth.

Why do we withdraw narcotics abruptly rather than decreasing them gradually to avoid the symptoms of withdrawal? In our experience, gradual withdrawal has been far less successful than abrupt withdrawal. Just as with any other addiction, such as smoking, the first step is a conscious decision to stop and a clear-cut act to end the addiction. We have found that symptoms of abrupt withdrawal are generally tolerable. On the other hand, if the patient has any symptoms, even in gradual withdrawal, he strives for just 'a little more' to prevent the dysphoria. This puts him back on a demand or reinforcement schedule which further potentiates the pain behavior. The best way to terminate the addiction is to terminate the narcotic.

That may be fine for a Chronic Pain Unit where the patients are in a controlled environment, but what about the doctor in office practice? The primary obligation of the physician in office practice is to recognize the ineffectiveness of analgesics as well as their danger, and to prevent the patient from getting into the addiction-withdrawal cycle in the first place. Tell the patient that there is no drug that will cure his pain. Television commercials to the contrary, there are conditions for which the best treatment is nothing at all. Patients will accept that if told directly by the physician and will cooperate with a withdrawal program. The doctor who jumps from one medication to another, gradually escalating the strength as well as the dose, is leading both himself and his patient into a dead end. Remember, patients find themselves in this position because well intentioned physicians prescribed the drugs for them.

What can an office practitioner do once a patient has entered the addiction-withdrawal cycle? Most patients can be taken off satisfactorily as outpatients if the following attitudes are present: (1) motivation on the part of the patient, (2) motivation on the part of the physician, (3) understanding of the program by both the patient and the physician, (4) sufficient fortitude to stick it out, despite craving for medication.

The patient might do well to spend the time with an intelligent, similarly motivated family member or friend who can provide needed moral support during the withdrawal period. Most patients with iatrogenic addiction have had a ceiling put on their dosages somewhere along the line (unless they are obtaining prescriptions from more than one physician), so their withdrawal is not likely to be as intense or dramatic as that of a street junkie.

What can be done about the patient who is taking such large doses of narcotics that abrupt withdrawal might not be safe, or the patient who has other medical problems that might contraindicate withdrawal? Patients whose dosage is dangerously high can be taken off narcotics with relative ease if the dose is decreased each day by 10–15% of the initial dose, so that withdrawal is complete in 7–10 days. The medicine should be prescribed by schedule and not on a prn basis. It must be stressed that the physician is in charge of the dosage schedule and that the patient is to take the medication only and exactly as prescribed. There is no extra medication, even if the pain becomes severe. There is to be no manipulation of the dosage schedule by the patient (or by the physician, for that matter). Each dose is to be given on the prescribed schedule, whether or not the patient needs it at that time, and no medication is to be given at any other time. When the schedule of medication administration is not dependent on the complaint of pain, most patients can be taken off narcotics successfully.

Some narcotic withdrawal is better managed in the hospital. Again, significant motivation is necessary, not only on the part of the patient and physician but also on the part of all of the nurses and hospital personnel involved with the patient's care. They must all recognize what is being done, since the usual philosophy is to medicate hospitalized patients when they have pain, which would be counterproductive in this circumstance.

It may be desirable to introduce into the program a process to remove the conditioning effects or positive reinforcement associated with the periodic administration of narcotics. In addition to the physiologic addiction that is associated with chronic administration of narcotics, each dose of narcotic psychologically reinforces further administration of narcotics, and in doing so, reinforces the chronic pain which justifies further administration of the drug. In essence, *the patient is being rewarded with the narcotic for having pain.* This behavior is well recognized in experimental animals who work extremely hard to get a reward of a shot of narcotic. It does not take too much extrapolation to perceive that pain patients undergo a similar conditioning process wherein the 'task' is to have pain and the 'reward' is the narcotic.

The conditioning and positive reinforcement associated with chronic administration of narcotics must be eliminated, since they are potent factors in the continuation of chronic pain. The only way to eliminate the reinforcement secondary to drug administration is to stop the drug. Such a plan coincides very nicely with the plan to alleviate narcotic addiction by abrupt discontinuation of the medication.

How might one deal with a patient whose psychological addiction is so great that compliance with a voluntary withdrawal program is unlikely? 'Plan A', as we call it, involves bringing the patient into the hospital where medication can be completely controlled. All medication is administered in quinine or other bitter tasting carrier, which serves as a negative reinforcement. Doses are given every 4 h around the clock, and the patient is awakened at night as scheduled. No prn medications are given at all. The daily dose of narcotics, as well as other medications, is determined from an accurate history. The same or slightly more narcotic equivalent is given in divided doses of methadone, which is one of the few narcotics absorbed when given orally. The patient is told that the initial daily dose is the same or somewhat greater than the amount of medication he had been taking, and he is also told that the medication dosage will thereafter be altered without informing him. The initial dose of medication is given for 2 or 3 days. The daily dose is then decreased by 15%, and by that same amount on subsequent days until, at the end of about a week, no narcotics at all are administered. During the time in which the dosage of medication is decreasing, the patient still receives quinine every 4 h, even if it contains no medication.

It is extremely helpful to keep the personnel on the floor blinded to the amount of medication in the quinine. If the patient is sure that he can get no information by asking, he will not hound the floor personnel to try to find out what dose he is receiving. We have an arrangement with the pharmacy so that the pharmacist and the prescribing physician alone know the dosage schedule.

Because of the bitter tasting carrier, the administration of medication constitutes negative reinforcement, rather than the positive reinforcement the patient had been receiving up to that time. In fact, patients often request that the 2.00 a.m. dose be omitted after the third or fourth day. After the patient has been receiving the carrier with no narcotic at all for several days, he can be told and the doses of quinine discontinued. It is surprising that patients may request that they continue to receive the quinine, knowing full well that there is no medication in it, but hanging on to the last symbolic vestige of medication ritual.

Our experience with narcotic analgesics in chronic pain patients can be summarized very simply:

1. Analgesics are not the answer to chronic pain.

2. Analgesics potentiate chronic pain.

3. Discontinuation of analgesics will break up the pattern of recurrent withdrawal, that is, the withdrawal-pain-narcotic-withdrawal cycle, which potentiates and intensifies the chronic pain.

4. Discontinuation of analgesics will eliminate positive reinforcement for pain behavior, which enhances the chronic pain.

5. Analgesics don't work for chronic pain, anyway!

b) Barbiturates

Barbiturates are often initially prescribed as sleeping aids for patients whose chronic pain may keep them awake. Unfortunately, the sleep induced by barbiturate administration differs from physiologic sleep in that it is deficient in REM periods and results in inadequate rest.

In addition, barbiturates, like narcotics, are highly addicting and rapidly produce tolerance. They take over the sleep regulating function of the brain so that after a few nights the patient begins to find that he cannot sleep without the barbiturates. An additional side-effect of chronic barbiturate administration is depression, which adds significantly to the depression already present in many chronic pain patients.

Because the patient has so much difficulty sleeping after the barbiturate has been discontinued, and because both the patient and the physician feel the compulsive need to 'do something', one barbiturate after another is substituted in an attempt to find some way that the patient can sleep. The substitution of nonbarbiturate sedatives is often futile and short-lived, since other sedatives do not prevent the symptoms of barbiturate withdrawal.

Again, the only way to alleviate the symptoms of barbiturate withdrawal is to discontinue the barbiturates. It is important that barbiturates *not* be discontinued abruptly, since seizures might result!

If the patient is taking the equivalent of 100 mg of pentobarbital at bedtime and no other barbiturates, withdrawal might be attempted on an outpatient basis. However, if the patient is taking barbiturates in doses larger than that, hospitalization is recommended, since the symptoms of barbiturate withdrawal can be severe and hazardous.

The major symptom of the withdrawal period about which the patient will complain vigorously is that of sleeplessness. The patient may be agitated for days during the period of withdrawal and a normal sleep pattern may not be instituted for several weeks. During that time, there is considerable fatigue and resultant craving for the barbiturate. Relaxation training and much encouragement may help the patient during this phase. The difference in the feelings and attitude of the patient who finally is no longer addicted makes the withdrawal process worthwhile.

In contrast to the withdrawal plan advocated for narcotics, the plan for barbiturate discontinuation should emphasize gradual withdrawal. Overabrupt withdrawal may result in a toxic psychosis or seizures. Generally, a safe rate of withdrawal is to decrease the initial daily dose by 15%, and to decrease the daily dose by that same amount every 2 days, so that the withdrawal period extends over 2 weeks.

There is no simple way to alleviate the insomnia that marks that period. However, coupling the withdrawal process with counseling and relaxation training will provide the patient with emotional support and perhaps considerable rest during this time.

c) Tranquilizers

The main problem with the use of tranquilizers for chronic pain patients is that they are often prescribed in place of psychological evaluation and counseling for emotional problems related to the chronic pain problem. Although tranquilizers may be extremely helpful for the management of transient periods of agitation, they do not take the place of a more definitive course of action. Consequently, they are best left to be prescribed by the psychiatrist or the individual counseling the patient, rather than being given independent of any other consideration.

When given on a chronic basis, however, most tranquilizers, especially the minor tranquilizers, contribute to the depression which is a hallmark of the chronic pain state. The use of major tranquilizers, when not specifically indicated for psychiatric disease, exposes patients to significant risks of neurological impairment, such as tardive dyskinesias, and the severe and involuntary movements of the extremities may persist even after the tranquilizers are discontinued.

Tranquilizers can be helpful for brief periods during the acute care phase of treatment after an injury. They can help the patient rest without narcotics. They can provide some relief from the tension and agitation that accompany musculoskeletal injuries and that may perpetuate the attendant muscle spasm.

However, when the patient is undergoing counseling for chronic pain and trying to readjust his attitudes and orientation so that he might be better able to cope with pain and minimize disability, the effects of tranquilizers can be counterproductive. At that time it is necessary for the patient to have full use of his intellectual and emotional resources in order to mount an optimal offensive against his chronic problem, and these powers are blunted significantly by tranquilizers. Consequently, we recommend that tranquilizers also be discontinued when the patient enters a program for the management of chronic pain.

Most tranquilizers can be discontinued abruptly with few side-effects except for the feeling of anxiety and agitation that the patient experiences temporarily. The exception is diazepam (Valium), which should be tapered gradually since overabrupt discontinuation of this medication may precipitate seizures, particularly in susceptible patients.

As with other medications, it must be recognized that long-term administration of tranquilizers does not usually contribute to the management of chronic pain, and may be counterproductive in the milieu of a comprehensive chronic pain program. Therefore, we recommend discontinuation of all tranquilizers, except in those patients for whom they are indicated for specific psychiatric reasons.

We have been stressing the overmedication prevalent among pain patients and the importance of discontinuing their medications. There are, however, two classes of medication that we have found helpful in treatment of chronic pain problems. They are the tricyclic antidepressants and the minor analgesics.

Tricyclic Antidepressants. The drug group that we have found the most useful in chronic pain patients is the tricyclic antidepressants. Almost all patients admitted to the Chronic Pain Unit receive these drugs. The two best known and most commonly administered are imipramine and amitriptyline. These drugs are specifically antidepressant and not stimulants. Their efficacy is clinically established in depression and there is also evidence that they raise pain threshold. Recommended dosage range for imipramine and amitriptyline is 25–150 mg per day for outpatients and 50–300 mg per day for inpatients. There is a lag of 3–21 days from time of first administration to time of clinical effect, so that if the patient has not responded after 3 weeks one must consider either discontinuing the medication or trying an alternate. Usual dosage schedule starts with 25 mg three times per day with 25 mg added to the nighttime dose until the patient reaches the maximum dosage for either the hospital or outpatient regimen. The dose is then decreased to minimal effective dosage, using drug tolerance and clinical response as guides. We have found the usual dosage to be 75–150 mg per day. The entire dose may be given at bedtime to minimize the sedative effects during the day and to help the patient re-establish a normal sleep cycle.

Side-effects of these antidepressants are extensions of their pharmacological action. The anti-cholinergic actions of the antidepressants may lead to blurred vision, dry mouth, urinary retention, paralytic ileus, and aggravation of acute angle glaucoma. Patients may also experience toxic delirium. On rare occasions patients will develop choliostatic jaundice. Antidepressants also tend to deplete the myocardium of catecholamines by preventing their reuptake, which can lead to unspecific T-wave changes and a potential for cardiac rhythm and conduction problems. Particularly in patients over 40, it is wise to have a baseline electrogram and to follow the patient's cardiovascular status.

Minor Analgesics. Patients who have arthritic, inflammatory or myositic components to their pain may benefit from the chronic use of minor analgesics such as salicylates, acetaminophen and phenacetin. The salicylates appear to be most effective against diffuse pain of low intensity, particularly that of inflammatory origin. They are suitable for chronic administration because there are no apparent long-term adverse effects and the acute adverse effects are well-known. Gastric irritation which may lead to ulceration and hemorrhage is common. Less appreciable, painless bleeding is seen occasionally with low dosages and can result in iron deficiency anemia. Prolonged bleeding induced by alteration in platelet adhesiveness is similarly associated with low dose usage.

Acetaminophen and phenacetin are analgesics with very weak anti-inflammatory effects. These drugs are very similar and are usually viewed as alternates to salicylates. Acetaminophen is preferred to phenacetin because it produces fewer unwanted reactions and is less toxic. Toxicity is primarily from overdose. A drug interaction of clinical concern is prolongation of the effect of oral anti-coagulants that can occur with chronic administration of full doses of acetaminophen.

Avoidance of Placebos. Before turning to the role of medication we would like to warn again against the use of placebo medication. The ineffectiveness and hazard of placebo trial for the differential diagnosis of chronic versus acute organic pain have been discussed. Even the saline 'mock block' (where the substitution of saline for anesthetic is made to predict therapy success or failure rather than to differentiate chronic from acute pain) must be interpreted with care.

Placebos have been improperly advocated for the diagnosis of chronic pain on the completely bogus assumption that acute organic pain will not be relieved by placebo, whereas pain with a large psychological component may be. Research documents the opposite. In controlled studies using subjects with severe acute or long-term pain who were administered placebo, pain relief occurred in 35% of subjects with 'real' pain. Powerful analgesics were found to be effective in only 75% of the cases, so placebos were about one-half as effective as active drugs. *Evans* refers to several studies which indicate that, where a placebo works, it is about 50% as effective as the analgesic it replaces.

Based, perhaps, upon such evidence, some physicians try placebo therapy on the chance that a given patient will respond, especially where active drugs are potentially addictive. These same studies, however, demonstrate that placebo is not a defensible alternative in management of chronic pain. First, test subjects generally receive one or two doses of placebo for acute, often severe, pain. Long-term effects of placebo have not been adequately tested, but it must be remembered that even active analgesics do not themselves provide significant relief from most chronic pain. Because placebo appears to derive its efficacy from the patient's expectations that an active pain killer is being administered and since the patient's long-lived pain has resisted all types of analgesics, placebo replacement cannot reasonably be expected to modify the pain in the long run.

The chief disservice of placebo treatment is its perpetuation of pill-taking, and therefore, sick role, behavior. The symbolic value of the pill has been discussed. A prescription means 'I am sick' to the patient and, moreover, prescription for an 'analgesic' means the pain is what is wrong and needs curing. This is the attitude that must be reversed by redefinition and the rehabilitation program. Studies show that the physician's belief in the potency of the prescription (be it drug or placebo) and enthusiastic endorsement of it are essential to its efficacy. Such belief is incompatible with our understanding of the true complex nature of the chronic pain syndrome. Perhaps most important, the patient's trust in the physician may be irretrievably shattered when the use is discontinued.

There is a broader 'placebo effect', however, which can derive from the doctor-patient relationship and which is independent of pill-taking. The physician's interest and strong suggestion as well as the patient's expectations for help are powerful components of the clinical milieu. With chronic pain patients, the potential of this beneficial placebo effect may be diminished by the unsatisfying treatment history and 'pain games'. Physicians must nonetheless exhibit the concern, encouragement and belief in the rehabilitation program that are the cornerstones of successful management.

C. Control of Pain Perception

Although it is generally not possible to control the underlying etiology of pain, it is helpful to combine a technique for the control of pain perception with the remainder of the comprehensive program. Some of these techniques are occasionally helpful when used alone, but their success rate improves markedly when they become part of an integrated program.

We have made passing reference to several modalities for the control of pain perception that may have a place in the management of chronic pain patients. Some can be carried out by the patient under the direction or tutelage of the primary care physician. These include relaxation training, support group activity, and transcutaneous stimulation. While each of these should not be considered as primary interventions, one or more of these techniques may be beneficial adjuncts to the total rehabilitation program.

1. Relaxation Training

Anxiety and tension play a large role in decreasing pain tolerance and increasing pain perception. Consequently, those techniques which help the patient learn to control anxiety and tension, such as relaxation training and biofeedback, also help the patient control pain perception. Moreover, such techniques allow the patient to sleep and relax without recourse to pharmacologic agents and their deleterious side-effects. Finally, it is well recognized that one side-effect of relaxation is diminished perception of pain.

A method for progressively relaxing the various muscles of the body until the entire body is relaxed or tension-free was introduced by *Edmund Jacobson* in 1929. Since then the technique has been found to aid in the treatment of such problems as anxiety, stress, insomnia, hypertension, asthma and headache. Its potential for controlling perception of chronic pain is two-fold. First, because tension, anxiety and stress figure so significantly in pain complaints, relaxation alone can often reduce the pain experience. Many people, others as well as pain patients, react to stress with narrowed focus on bodily concerns, exaggerated perception of existing organic symptoms and tension (see Chapter IV). Restrictions in normal body movement made to favor painful areas can also add to muscle tension and fatigue. The poor muscle tone and limited activity tolerance which accompany the physical inactivity of the regressed state also contribute to the problem. Muscle tension, painful in itself, elaborates existing pain. Where proper relaxation is achieved, muscle tension, anxiety, and general arousal-producing input decrease. In a completely relaxed state, anxiety and attention to bodily concerns disappear; *Jacobson* refers to this state as 'going negative'.

The resemblance between the relaxed state and hypnotic trance has long been recognized. Physiological similarities between the two (decreased oxygen consumption, respiration and heart rate, increased alpha waves on EEG, and others) lead some to equate relaxation with neutral hypnosis. When deeper trance is desired for suggestion of analgesia, relaxation is almost exclusively the mode of induction. The second possible use for relaxation in pain control, then, is its service as a technique for induction of hypnosis.

Jacobson's method for teaching relaxation begins with the instruction first to tense, then to relax given muscle groups throughout the body. The tensing is a very important part of the procedure. The patient tenses the given muscles until fatigue can be felt in those and connected muscles and then relaxes, feeling the tension disappearing.

Relaxation is a motor skill that is learned like other such skills, at varying speeds and with varying degrees of required practice by different individuals. Because of this, it has recently been found convenient to tape the instructions so patients can practice at home. Many commercially available tapes contain the initial 15- to 30-minute instructions on one side of the tape, with a shorter version on the other for those who have progressed farther. *Ferguson* and his co-workers note, however, that many patients prefer their own physician's voice on the tape and have therefore prepared 'A Script for Deep Muscle Relaxation' which can be read and recorded by the physician.

2. Support Group Meetings

By support groups we do not mean group psychotherapy, but meetings among peers for mutual support. As we have said, the majority of chronic pain patients are convinced they are ill and resist attempts to define their problems in psychological terms. Furthermore, many share an inability to recognize symptoms of stress and conflict as emotional events but express these discomforts as somatic complaints. For these reasons, traditional insight and interpretive group psychotherapy are beyond the interest and capability of many chronic pain patients. Individual psychotherapy, with the few for whom it is useful, is not to be thought of as a pain control treatment.

Group discussions between patients with similar problems, with or without a therapist but preferably without a physician, have been found to provide several valuable services. Chief among these are support, education, and a means of re-entry into responsible social interaction. The opportunity for support from those with similar problems but at various stages of rehabilitation is obvious. Peers accept and encourage. They also confront fellow patients who backslide into familiar pain games. More advanced group members can see their real progress in comparison to newcomers and take further reinforcement from their status as helpers.

Education in the group may include dissemination of medical information, but should focus on role redefinition and the issues raised by abandonment of the acute sick role. Concerns over resuming marital, family, social, occupational, or financial responsibilities are common to all and, again, the experience of the more fully resocialized members is invaluable. The cause of re-education is often advanced by not having a physician participant. It has been found that where a physician is present, patients revert to using medical problems as a means for social interaction and attempt to re-establish an inappropriate doctor-patient relationship. The groups are often more effective when organized and maintained by rehabilitated patients under the direction of paraprofessionals.

As a means for facilitating re-entry into the role of healthy adult or into an adapted normal role, support groups can have widespread influence. They can be critical in helping patients transfer to daily home life the well behaviors and skills learned during an inpatient stay. As a form of social interaction, support groups make social responsibility demands of their members and promote resocialization. At the same time, the protected and sympathetic environment reduces the risk associated with resuming an unused (or for some, assuming a brand new) role. Support groups, directing attention away from patienthood and toward family and social concerns, discourage the use of pain as a means of establishing or avoiding interpersonal relationships. This is a most important intermediate step between sick role occupancy and re-entry into the role of normal adult.

3. Transcutaneous Stimulation

There has been a great deal of both information and misinformation about transcutaneous stimulation (TENS) in the literature in recent years. Transcutaneous stimulation is the administration of an electrical stimulus to the skin. The stimulator is a battery-operated unit about the size of a pack of cigarettes, which can be worn clipped to the belt or inconspicuously inside the clothes. It is attached by means of lead wires to either two or four electrodes that are taped to the skin. The electrodes are usually rubberized thin pads, the size of which varies according to the area to be stimulated. The patient adjusts the voltage so that the sensation is perceptible but not painful. The stimulator can be used constantly or intermittently, depending on the response of the patient.

Several theories are offered to explain the effectiveness of transcutaneous stimulation. The simplest, expressed by many unsophisticated, but perhaps quite perceptive, patients, is that 'it takes my mind off the pain'. Certainly diversional therapy is valuable in chronic pain states, and that may indeed by one key to the success of transcutaneous stimulation.

More likely, influence on the Melzack-Wall gate is involved. The gate theory, remember, holds that non-painful sensation competes with and inhibits painful sensation through a system of mutually interacting neurons at each segmental level of the spinal cord. When a non-painful stimulus is applied, it literally inhibits the perception of pain by closing the gate and blocking the transmission of a painful stimulus at spinal cord levels. The simplest and most physiologic demonstration of this is 'when you rub it, it hurts less'. It is almost instinctively recognized that, very often, rubbing a painful area decreases the pain. Rubbing, of course, stimulates the large nerve fibers which are involved with the perception of non-painful stimulation. According to the gate theory, the stimulation of such fibers inhibits the firing of those neurons that transmit pain. Since it is not feasible to walk around all day rubbing the part that hurts, a more scientific approach has been taken. The application of an electrical stimulus to the surface of the skin produces a similar result. Because the large neurons concerned with the perception of non-painful information have a lower threshold than pain neurons, they are stimulated first as the voltage is gradually increased, and the patient perceives the stimulus to be non-painful. It is only when the voltage increases above the threshold for the smaller fibers that the sensation is perceived as being painful. Thus, by definition, when the patient regulates the voltage so that he perceives the sensation, but it is not painful, he is stimulating those large neurons which, according to the gate theory, inhibit pain sensation.

We have found transcutaneous stimulation to be a helpful modality in approximately one-half of the patients on whom we have used it. Several factors influence the success or failure of the procedure.

(1) The effectiveness of transcutaneous stimulation increased significantly when employed with patients who do not have the many psychosocial concomitants of chronic pain discussed here. It is much less effective in patients who are depressed, anxious or agitated. In fact, the 'bother' of caring for any stimulation device may add to the agitation of such patients, so that chronic stimulation of any kind is contraindicated in depression or agitation.

(2) Transcutaneous stimulation is much more successful when incorporated into a comprehensive program than when used alone.

(3) Transcutaneous stimulation is for symptomatic control only. If there is a progressive underlying etiology, the patient's pain may break through the effect of the stimulation.

(4) It takes a great deal of time and work with the patient to establish a successful program of transcutaneous stimulation. Contrary to the unrealistic hopes of many clinicians, you cannot write a prescription for a transcutaneous stimulator and consider that the patient has been treated. Several hours are usually required to instruct the patient about the use of the stimulator, allow him to get to the point at which he feels comfortable and secure about using an electronic device, and establish the optimal sites of electrode placement.

Either a single channel (two electrodes) or a dual channel (four electrodes) stimulator can be employed, depending on the extent of the pain. The electrodes may be applied initially to the area of the pain or across the area of the pain. Trial application of the electrodes should be made adjacent to the pain, particularly in the same dermatome. An occasional patient will obtain relief from electrodes applied to the contralateral side of the body in the mirror-image area of the pain. Whatever appeals most to the patient and whatever affords the patient the best pain relief is the optimal position. There is no magic formula, nor is there any single electrode placement that is guaranteed to work. There is nothing that takes the place of spending time with the patent, reassuring him, and seeking optimal use of the transcutaneous stimulator through patient trial and error.

Because we have found transcutaneous stimulation to be so helpful in a multitude of various types of pain problems, we recommend that family physicians in general should familiarize themselves with its use.

D. Remobilization

This section is short, not because remobilization is not important, but because it is such a basic part of any chronic pain program that it can be discussed simply and efficiently.

A necessary prerequisite to remobilization is patient motivation, which can be enhanced by participation in the rest of the comprehensive program.

Remobilization is part of the resocialization procedure. It changes the orientation of physician advice to the patient from 'Don't ...' to 'Do more'. It involves increasing physical activity in a graduated manner that the patient can tolerate, so that he can eventually regain sufficient physical activity to overcome the disability state. The remobilization program is intended to combat the excessive immobilization which characterizes most chronic patients, many of them acting on the advice of their physician, and to avoid the erratic swings in amount of physical activity a patient might undertake on his own.

Apart from disease itself, most patients are in poor general health and physical condition secondary to their excessive inactivity and disability. A regimen of general productive activity leading to an exercise program should be instituted. Specific exercises should be prescribed to strengthen the individual's surgery or injury site, the low back, for example. It should be explained to the patient that these, in themselves, will not relieve pain; they are intended to prevent the vulnerability to further injury that inactivity promotes.

When a patient presents with an acute problem it is perfectly appropriate for the physician to instruct the patient to rest in anticipation that the acute problem will resolve and the patient will resume activities. When pain has become chronic and spontaneous remission can no longer be anticipated, rest is often not the appropriate recommendation.

Unfortunately, many physicians do not make the distinction between acute and chronic pain management. The patient complains of pain and an automatic recommendation to rest follows. The patient notes on successive visits that certain activities make the pain worse, and receives instructions to decrease his activity further. As a result, the patient becomes increasingly immobilized, but rarely more pain free.

It is amazing how many patients arrive at the Pain Clinic with a long list of 'don'ts', but admit that their doctor never indicated what they *could* do. The usual result of such negative advice is that the patient becomes more and more fearful of doing anything at all. The fear enhances the patient's tension and anxiety, which further contribute to distress.

If one were to put a perfectly healthy individual in bed for 6 months, that individual would find resumption of even modest activity to be painful. During that time his muscles would have become so atrophic, tight, and out of shape that normal activity would constitute extreme physical stress that would provoke fatigue and pain. Yet we commit pain patients to prolonged periods of inactivity or bedrest and are then surprised when they are unable to get out of bed to do anything.

Patients are frequently aware of that phenomenon and will use it to justify their disability. The classic example is the patient who spent 6 months in bed after having suffered an injury on the job and had minimal activity thereafter. One day he decided to mow the lawn. Although he did not feel pain immediately, he 'paid for it' for 3 days after that, and had to stay in bed during that time. Certainly this story has the (consciously or unconsciously) desired effect of *proving* that the patient is incapable of physical activity. It seems curious that male patients so often select mowing the lawn as their trial of vigorous activity, and women select vacuuming the house. Both of these activities involve pushing, pulling and twisting motions with inefficient leverages of the back and are well designed to stress the musculoskeletal system, particularly one that is not in good shape.

Immobilization is a characteristic part of the regression which accompanies chronic pain. The answer to immobilization is, logically, remobilization, and this is a key factor in overcoming regression and consequently one of the major aspects of the comprehensive pain treatment program.

The keys to remobilization are that it should be (1) gradual and (2) progressive.

When physical activity is first resumed, patients may feel an increase in pain. They have been told so often to avoid *any* activity which would cause pain that they would need guidance and reassurance. We tell patients that the initial increase in activity will cause a 'spring training' effect. The athlete expects to hurt after the first day of spring training. His response is not to retire and stop exercising, but to come back for another day of training. By the end of the first week, the pain gives way to a feeling of well being and vigor.

Patients are no different, but their level of activity is much lower and their rate of progress slower. In contrast to the athlete, they enter the physical activity in anticipation of failure, and require considerable encouragement and reinforcement. Activity levels must be geared to the individual patient and clinical problem. The first step is to discourage inactivity. The patient should be instructed to get out of bed in the morning, get dressed and not return to bed or to the reclining position until bedtime that night. If it is not possible for the patient to be up all of the first day, he should follow a schedule designed by the physician which calls for his being up longer each day and leads to his staying up all day within a few days. Initial physical activities should be those required for self-care. Not only does this promote movement of the body, but it is a step toward independence and away from regression.

When the patient can be up most or all of the day, a program of gradually progressive exercises can be initiated. It is important to begin at a level that the patient can manage, and to allow progression toward vigorous physical exertion at the patient's own rate. Successful remobilization may take several months. Combined with physical activity, counseling and resocialization, it is one of the mainstays of any chronic pain program.

The Williams' flexion exercises are those most often prescribed by many physicians for patients with chronic low back problems. We find that many patients have difficulty with the sit-ups, and that the program is neither as flexible nor infinitely progressive as one might wish. We have had somewhat better luck with the 'Royal Canadian Air Force Exercise Plan for Physical Fitness', which is available as an inexpensive manual in most bookstores. All patients should start at the very first level, and they should progress quite slowly. It is important to exercise every day. Running in place is perhaps too vigorous for chronic pain patients, but walking can be substituted.

The second key to remobilization is progression – 'every day a little bit more'. Patients need frequent encouragement. They will have to have their programs monitored to assess whether any activity is contraindicated because of specific mechanical difficulties. Contraindications should be few and patients should be encouraged to do everything possible. Positive recommendations should be emphasized, and negative recommendations kept to a minimum.

The goals for remobilization should be identified reasonably soon after the patient begins the program. This allows the patient to see where he is going, and be encouraged as each successive goal is reached. The ultimate goal is for the patient to return to the level of activity required for participation in those jobs and pastimes which provide gratification. The goal of remobilization, in other words, is the goal of the overall program. For some patients, that may mean only a return to self-care or care with minimal help. For other patients, it may mean a return to recreational activities. For still others, it may represent return to gainful employment.

It is important that the level of remobilization coincides with vocational demands if the patient's goal is to return to work. It is often overlooked that some jobs require a great deal of physical activity that is possible only because a physical conditioning process has taken place over many years of working. When the individual is away from the physical activity, even for a few days or a few weeks, the conditioning process reverses, and it may be quite difficult for him to return to work. If this situation is compounded by a chronic pain state, it is almost certain that the patient will have an increase in pain upon returning to a physically demanding occupation. The patient should be allowed to increase physical activity gradually to the point that the physical demands of the job can be met *prior* to an attempt to return to work. The physician should work with the patient to devise an exercise program which can be carried out on a regular basis and which will include progressive activity of the kind required by employment. This may take the form of walking progressing to running. It may take the form of stair-climbing progressing to ladder climbing. It may take the form of weight-lifting, starting with bending, progressing to very light weights which present no challenge and then to weights comparable to those handled on the job.

The remobilization program must be tailored to the goals and activities of each individual patient. There is no set formula, except for the gradual and progressive nature of any program employed. Any physician who takes the time to guide the patient to realistic goals should be able to devise a progressive program to attain these goals.

E. Specific Treatment

At one time, it was naively thought that chronic pain could be treated merely by interrupting the pathway commonly associated with the transmission of acute pain. Although it appeared logical at the time, long experience has demonstrated that procedures to ablate pain pathways rarely produce prolonged relief of chronic pain. Although such procedures have been found extremely useful in the treatment of cancer pain, they are virtually useless for chronic pain.

Recommendations for many specific therapies for pain appear regularly in the literature and disappear just as regularly. There is considerable disagreement about the effectiveness of many therapies, whether they be stimulation, blocks, physical modalities, drugs, or even magic. Many of the reasons for the disagreement become apparent when one looks at the pattern by which a pain procedure is accepted.

The initial report is usually based on just a few cases. If a treatment is unsuccessful in the first few cases, it is forgotten and the report never published, so treatments reported in the literature are selected with a bias for early successes. One must recognize that given enough trials the success rate may have been the same in both published and forgotten studies, but with so few experimental cases there is an excellent statistical possibility that similar outcomes – successful or unsuccessful – will coincidentally occur together at first. One factor which promotes success is the magical effect of being the first patient to try an 'experimental' procedure. Both the physician and patient are hoping for success and the fame that results, for the former in scientific circles, and for the latter at the local bridge club. A related predisposition to success in the first few trials stems from the investigator's enthusiasm for his own brain-child. If he were not enthusiastic, he would not have pursued it.

Many patients with chronic pain have in their histories a string of temporary successes from an assortment of treatment programs. It may take 3–6 months before a failure becomes apparent and then patient disillusionment is often reported to a different physician. These temporary successes may be prematurely reported as successes by the investigator. Moreover, concern that someone else may stumble across the same treatment and publish first provides additional pressure to produce an enthusiastic first report promptly.

The initial report may be so enthusiastic, possibly even recording total pain relief in all patients, that no other investigator can duplicate the success. Follow-up investigators become disenchanted, and their disenchantment is readily felt by their patients. A string of reports of failures follows in the literature. Meanwhile, the original investigator's delayed failures are beginning to catch up to him. He begins to doubt his original findings, and, as his enthusiasm wanes, less patient acceptance leads to a lower success rate.

After the extreme positive and the extreme negative reports appear, a small group of tenacious, objective investigators may continue to evaluate this new treatment, recognizing that it provides modest success in a limited group of patients. They may or may not learn how to identify this group of patients in advance but are content to employ the procedure with appropriate reservation. The use of the procedure with restrained enthusiasm may then level off or it may be forgotten in the literature, only to be rediscovered with the same initial enthusiasm 15 years later. This appears to be the time during which the generation that witnessed the original debate has retired into a well-set routine, and the new generation of enthusiastic innovators is not familiar with the literature so far back. It is only after rediscovery that someone, usually one of the skeptics, discovers that this procedure is not new after all, but is one that was abandoned 15 years previously.

Thus, we can see the various external factors that influence the 'success' of a procedure – an investigator's contagious enthusiasm, the patient's resultant enthusiasm, the patient's wish to please the physician, other investigator's skepticism, either enthusiastic or negative reports in the literature, and the duration of follow-up. Added to these influences is the degree of magnetism of the investigator's personality. There are those colleagues whose personalities are so influential that anything they administer to patients is successful, at least temporarily. There are others whose personalities are so bland or negative that even the best modality is doomed to failure in their hands.

With chronic pain treatments there is the additional truth that most specific treatments for chronic pain exert a quantitative effect, that is, they may lessen the pain, but usually do not turn it off completely. The degree of pain relief is subject to the many variables in the patient's own personality and pain-disability state that were discussed in Chapter IV, including pre-existing personality, social pressures, financial rewards, family pressures, secondary gain, conditioned behavior, and the acceptance of disability behavior.

It is difficult to evaluate any modality for the treatment of pain in the midst of so many influences on pain perception and, consequently, on success of the treatment modality. In the face of the many psychological, medical, and social factors that encourage the patient to have pain, any treatment – no matter how logical – cannot be expected to make that pain go away. It is similarly unlikely that *any* specific therapy used in isolation would be successful against a complex multi-faceted chronic pain syndrome incorporating all of the physical and psychosocial factors already presented. The complex problem of pain deserves better than the simplistic treatment it gets in television advertising where neurotic people rid themselves of tension headaches by popping two pills.

If a patient's condition has not evolved into the complex chronic pain-disability state, temporary symptomatic therapy with one of the specific modalities discussed below may be helpful. If, however, the patient has progressed to the full-blown chronic pain syndrome described herein, it is extremely unlikely that a simple, single therapeutic technique will be successful. Once any modality has been tried unsuccessfully, even under the most unfavorable of circumstances, it is far less likely to be successful if used again later when the overall situation is better. Consequently, we recommend postponing specific treatment for pain in the chronic pain syndrome group until the patient is well established in a comprehensive program.

Some specific therapies are directed to the underlying etiology rather than to pain perception. Others, such as transcutaneous stimulation, affect pain perception and can be used regardless of the etiology, although they may be more effective for certain types of pain. Some therapies affect both. Physical therapy, for instance, may help control pain perception through counter-irritation and relaxation, but it is more importantly directed toward relaxing underlying muscle spasm or as an aid to remobilization.

As a general rule, we have virtually abandoned ablative procedures for the treatment of chronic pain of benign origin. These include peripheral neurectomy (either surgical or chemical), dorsal rhizotomy, cordotomy (either percutaneous or surgical), and procedures interrupting the pain pathways within the brain, but trigger point blocks are not considered under this category. Exceptions are extremely few and must be justified on the basis of specific etiology. Curiously, if chronic pain originates from an injury to a nerve, once the chronic pain has become established, interrupting that nerve or nerve root rarely provides long-term relief.

There have been many reports which hold a contrary viewpoint, that is, advocating increasingly refined methods of interrupting the classical pain pathway. Most of those procedures claim a 30–50% improvement in long-term follow-up, which is not far beyond the placebo effect one would expect. However, virtually all of them also report complications or side-effects which include pain or dysesthesia more severe than the pain originally being treated. Although it is difficult to evaluate pre-morbid personality in retrospect, it is our impression that the incidence of such post-denervation dysesthesia is particularly prevalent in those patients, described in Chapter IV, whose personalities indicate a need to suffer.

1. Biofeedback

Biofeedback is a technique of training the patient to become better able to control physiologic processes. The mechanism of its effectiveness in pain management is still undetermined, but evidence indicates that it can be particularly useful for relief of tension headaches and other muscular tension based pain problems. It can be useful in a broad-based pain treatment program by contributing significantly to the patient's ability to relax and by enabling the patient to overcome the feeling of helplessness that frequently accompanies the chronic pain state.

In biofeedback, a physiologic process is monitored and electronically displayed by either an auditory or visual signal. The patient attempts to reduce the activity of the monitored area consciously or to bring the activity to a predetermined level, and he is rewarded and encouraged by diminution or normalization of the biofeedback signal.

The theory behind biofeedback training holds that individuals can gain some control over autonomic, so-called involuntary, functions by being made immediately aware of changes in these processes, that is, through feedback of the biological activity. When the desired goal is achieved, such as muscle relaxation, a visual or auditory signal is presented to the patient. The immediate goal is production of the desired signal. If attainment of that goal brings relief from pain, the behavior which produced the change in the signal is reinforced. The eventual goal is achievement of a body state in which pain perception is reduced without electronic monitoring. Among visceral responses that have, under laboratory and clinical conditions, been altered with biofeedback training are heartbeat, blood pressure, muscle activity, surface skin temperature, and brain wave frequency.

Biofeedback training has been used for blood pressure or heart rate control, seizure control, gastrointestinal and cardiovascular disorders, and vascular headaches, as well as for chronic pain. It has been particularly successful in treating tension headache. As a tool in chronic pain management, biofeedback is probably most successful where pain is due to muscle spasm and tension.

Three types of biofeedback can be helpful. In one form, muscle activity is monitored from an area where tension or spasms is suspected. An electrode is attached at the site and the level of electromyographic muscle activity (EMG) is displayed. The patient is instructed to reduce the amount of activity in that muscle. This type of monitoring is particularly useful when the low back or posterior cervical muscles are involved. The patient learns to relax the painful muscles, thereby directly decreasing the pain. In tension headache or other tension states, the frontalis muscle or suboccipital muscle group is monitored, inasmuch as decreased activity there seems to reduce tension in the head, scalp, neck, and upper body muscles.

Curiously, the acquisition of ability to control almost any bodily function results in the ability to control tension, which provides additional opportunities for the development of feedback signals. One of the most commonly used signals is that of skin temperature, particularly of the hands or fingers. This is easy to monitor, and provides a signal which is easy to manipulate with biofeedback apparatus. A thermocouple is taped to a hand or finger, and the signal is led to a temperature sensing device. The patient is instructed to try to raise the temperature of the part, that is, to increase the blood supply to the area. Doing so establishes a state of relaxation, which may be particularly helpful for such conditions as tension headache or muscle spasm pain.

In a third form of biofeedback, the occipital EEG is used as the bio-feedback signal. Since alpha waves may dominate in periods of relaxation, the theory is that the voluntary assumption of the 'alpha state', i.e., alpha rhythm dominance, will lead to relaxation. The patient is presented a signal which represents alpha wave activity, rather than one which represents raw EEG data. The patient is asked to produce the alpha activity signal volun-tarily and, with practice, to maintain that state.

Researchers have found when comparing decreased pain perception after biofeedback training to relief from control (placebo) sessions, relax-ation sessions, and hypnosis, that biofeedback training adds to patients' ability to control pain perception. The most significant reduction of pain reported has been achieved by biofeedback training employed as an aid to relaxation or in tandem with strong suggestion or hypnosis. *Melzack* explains that alpha training combines aspects of placebo and relaxation with its own special ability to demand patient attention. It helps to maintain a 'meditational state' by (1) directing attention away from the painful body part and toward the feedback signal, (2) suggesting that the procedure will reduce pain, (3) aiding relaxation, and (4) providing subjects with a sense of voluntary control over pain, which belief, in itself, lowers the level of per-ceived pain.

The biofeedback monitor is used only as a training tool. The goal is for the patient to develop through practice sufficient control of the bodily function of interest so that he can control it even when it is not moni-tored.

The first phase of training is for the patient to receive the monitored signal and to make a conscious effort to alter that signal. The second stage is to bring the alteration of the signal to a predetermined level and consciously hold it at that level while being monitored. The third phase is attained when the patient is able to alter the body process in the intended manner even when it is not being monitored. The fourth phase and ultimate goal is incorporation of that alteration into the patient's repertoire of automatic behavior.

Long-term relief is as uncertain with a simple course of biofeedback as it is with other modalities discussed earlier. Transfer from a training envi-ronment to a home situation can wipe out early benefits. Home relaxation tapes, autogenic training, monthly group sessions and 'booster' feedback sessions are currently employed as 'transfer' procedures.

If a biofeedback laboratory is available in the area, biofeedback train-ing can be added to the patient's comprehensive pain program. It may be particularly helpful in patients with tension headache, myofascial syndrome or pain of muscular origin, but is only recommended as a part of an overall comprehensive program and not as a treatment in itself.

2. Physical Therapy

Physical therapy for chronic pain patients has three major related functions. The first general function ('Rub it and it feels better') is to provide counter-irritation or, more accurately, counter-stimulation, as a means of inhibiting pain perception (see the discussion of transcutaneous stimulation). The second general purpose ('Gee, that feels good') is to enable the patient to relax and derive benefit from the same mechanism that is at work in the relaxation training program. The third, more specific, effect is the alleviation of muscle tension and spasm when those factors are sources of pain.

The first effect, counter-stimulation, can be achieved in several ways. Local massage over the area of pain is the procedure of choice, and stimulates large low-threshold nerve fibers with non-painful sensation, so the resultant large nerve fiber input tends to close the gate or inhibit perception of pain. This appears to be more than simple competition and certainly more than merely distraction; it is a specific physiologic effect. There is a possibility that ultrasound or low-frequency stimulation produces similar counter-stimulation, even though the perception of cutaneous sensation may be minimal.

The application of heat or cold may likewise reduce muscle tension or spasm. Particularly with the application of heat there are added elements of relaxation. Either heat or cold may relieve local muscle spasm or inflammation. The patient is generally the best judge of which temperature provides more relief. Many patients will have already tried either, so that asking the patient whether he benefits from warm or cold applications is often the most efficient way to settle on the more valuable of the two treatments.

Deep heat is generally better than heat more superficially applied. In the Physical Therapy Department, it can be administered as infrared radiation or moist hot packs.

There is one program for the outpatient application of moist heat which is especially successful, particularly in patients with myofascial syndrome and a great deal of superimposed tension (whether they be chronic pain patients or not). The patient is instructed to sit in a tub of hot water for

30 minutes two or three times a day. He is to set aside specific times each day so as not to be interrupted. It is suggested that he take some relaxing reading material with him and remain immersed up to his chin. This provides deep penetrating heat to muscles which may be sore or in spasm, with the specific local effect of muscle relaxation and decrease in inflammation. It provides the counter-stimulation of the warm water, which can be intensified by use of a whirlpool system. Perhaps most important, it provides programmed relaxation at scheduled times during the day, when the patient can escape from tension-producing activities and remain secreted in a relaxing environment.

Ultrasound may, in addition to providing counter-stimulation, have a direct effect on muscles in spasm. It can be particularly helpful to those patients who have muscle strain or myofascial pain of the trunk or neck, and may also loosen tight extremities, especially when combined with muscle stretching exercises.

3. Blocks

We have already indicated that blocks may be of some diagnostic value, but their effect must be interpreted with caution. We have also noted that ablative procedures, including permanent peripheral nerve blocks, are rarely indicated for chronic pain of benign origin. (Ablative procedures, in general, can be of considerable value in managing patients with cancer pain, but that is beyond the scope of this treatise.)

Blocks of trigger points of myofascial syndrome can be of significant long-term benefit, particularly when part of a comprehensive chronic pain program. The technique for identifying trigger points and injecting these trigger points has already been explained (Chapter VIII, page 79). Once it has been established by the use of multiple trigger point injections that a patient obtains pain relief from trigger point blocks, a protocol for using blocks in a therapeutic manner can be instituted.

The initial procedure involves blocking with the trigger point several times with a local anesthetic, such as lidocaine, and progressing to a long-acting local anesthetic, such as bupivicaine. During the time that the local anesthetic is in effect, gentle active and passive range of motion exercises can be employed in order to stretch the shortened muscles in the painful area. The patient should be cautioned that such a maneuver might cause a temporary flare-up in the pain, and if this becomes too severe exercising may have to be temporarily cut back.

When the specific trigger points have been identified, they may be marked on the skin in ink. Each point is then injected individually after the skin has been wiped with antiseptic. We prefer to use a 22 gauge, 1½ inch needle. Care must be taken to assure that the tip of the needle is inserted to the proper plane, usually at the insertion of muscle or just deep to the lumbodorsal fascia or ligamentum nuchae. The patient usually reports promptly when the needle has entered the trigger point. The trigger point is then injected with 1 cm^3 of lidocaine for local anesthesia.

If pain persists despite four or five local anesthetic blocks, a corticosteroid such as triamcinolone may be incorporated into the local anesthetic in hopes of decreasing the local inflammatory reaction that potentiates trigger point pain. This combination of injections may furnish long-lasting relief, but should not be given more often than every 3 or 4 days for a maximum of 3 weeks. Attention must be given to the total dose of steroid administered, since it is absorbed systemically and can lead to such common side-effects of steroid administration as ulcer disease, or a cushinoid state or pituitary suppression.

If the pain returns despite the program of multiple anesthetic and steroid blocks, relief can be made more permanent by the injection of alcohol or phenol. Although the alcohol diffuses more broadly than phenol, making it easier to hit a specific trigger point, it is more painful at the time of injection and may be followed by a more significant inflammatory response with exacerbation of pain. Consequently, we prefer phenol for well localized trigger points. Prior to embarking on a program of alcohol or phenol injection, the physician should warn patients that the injection may increase the pain temporarily, even if ultimately successful.

Phenol can be used in 5–10% solution. It is convenient to have the pharmacy make up vials of 500 mg of phenol crystals. The crystals can be diluted in 5–10 cm^3 of saline for injection to provide a sufficient strength of phenol in a sufficient volume for injection. No more than 2 cm^3 or 100 mg should be injected at any trigger point, and then only after the area has first been anesthetized.

The procedure begins as outlined for the diagnosis of trigger points. The area is palpated for tenderness, muscle spasm and/or nodularity. The most likely areas for trigger points, particularly in low back pain, are along the paravertebral muscles at the crest of the sacrum of ilium. Trigger points are frequently near incisions made for the purpose of stripping muscles from bone, as after laminectomy and/or fusion, and at the donor site of a fusion.

If phenol or alcohol is to be injected, the trigger point is first injected in the usual fashion. The needle is left in place, but the syringe is gently removed from it. A 5–10 cm³ syringe containing the phenol solution is attached to the needle and 1 or 2 cm³ is injected. The needle and syringe are then removed together, while gentle suction is maintained.

No more than five trigger points should be blocked at any one sitting. The injection should not be repeated too frequently because there is often a temporary increase in pain following the injection, and clinical results cannot be evaluated during that time. In each series, no more than five injections every 4–7 days is the maximum tolerated. As many as 15–20 trigger points can be gradually treated in this fashion. It may be necessary to treat each trigger point two or three times, particularly if the area of pain is broad.

Extreme caution should be exercised when blocking trigger points very near the spine or in the cervical area. Always aspirate very carefully to assure that cerebrospinal fluid or blood is not obtained. Do not inject if there is any possibility of epidural, subarachnoid or intravascular injection. Injection of an artery en route to the spinal cord can result in a spinal cord infarction and resultant quadriplegia or paraplegia.

When the patient has alleviation of pain immediately following each injection, the opportunity should be taken to improve mobility. Stretching exercises may be performed at that time, but they should be gentle so further tissue damage does not occur.

If pain returns several weeks or months following a series of trigger point injections, the entire series can be repeated. Meanwhile, however, the patient should be engaged in the resocialization and remobilization phases of the chronic pain program.

4. Hypnosis

Hypnosis has been compared not only to a state of relaxation, but to such other possible pain control mechanisms as brain wave control, acupuncture, placebo and meditation. In comparative studies, researchers differentiate between two hypnotic states – one very similar to the relaxation described on pages 106 and 117 called *neutral* or *relaxation hypnosis,* and the deep trance in which analgesia, anesthesia, regression in time and other 'tasks' can be accomplished through suggestion, often called task hypnosis. A larger percentage of the population can achieve neutral hypnosis while perhaps only 10–15% can reach the level necessary for full hypnoanesthesia. Both clinical and experimental study results concur that relaxation hypnosis can reduce perception of pain significantly more than control 'placebo' session where hypnosis is not induced. Physiologic responses to pain by hypnotized and nonhypnotized but relaxed subjects were often very similar, but the subjective report from hypnotized patients was of greater comfort and less pain.

Some evidence suggests that pain patients are less susceptible to hypnosis than a random group of research subjects. *Orne* contends that, among pain patients, those with severe organic pain like that of terminal cancer, for instance, get more relief than those with functional pain. Both statements are understandable in light of the point we have been making throughout – most chronic pain patients use pain as a way to avoid dealing with conflict and are reluctant to gain control over, or let go of, the pain before another resolution can be substituted. Consequently, control of pain by the techniques discussed here must be secondary to the primary goal – removal from the sick role.

We have not employed hypnosis routinely in our chronic pain program. We have found that *Jacobson's* relaxation techniques have provided most of the benefit that might have been obtained from formal hypnosis sessions at far less time commitment and expense. If a psychiatrist or psychologist skilled in hypnosis is available, hypnosis can be a valuable adjunct in selected patients. Particularly good candidates might be those with atypical facial pain, pain specifically related to tension states, or pain with associated tics in patients who do not respond to the usual program.

Where hypnosis is part of the rehabilitation program, patients are usually trained by the physician as they are in relaxation and given a tape for practicing at home. Eventually patients practice self-hypnosis independently. Follow-up reports show that some patients continue to find relief through hypnosis for months after training.

5. Acupuncture

The use of acupuncture for the treatment of chronic pain is controversial, poorly understood, and frequently abused. Nevertheless, in conservative and ethical hands, acupuncture has afforded pain relief for a few of our patients for whom we had no other answer.

A greater aura of mystery surrounds acupuncture, perhaps, than any of the other measures we have discussed. A period of unlimited claims and uncertain practices followed the popularization of acupuncture in the Western world several decades ago. More recently valid research and clinical reports have begun to confirm the analgesic capabilities of this ancient procedure.

Although the mechanism of acupuncture analgesia is unknown, there appears to be considerable basis for some physiologic effect. The increase in pain threshold in experimental animals as a result of acupuncture cannot be attributed to placebo or psychological effect.

In treatment by acupuncture, fine needles of silver, gold, or steel are inserted into specific points on the skin and may be manipulated or stimulated electrically for periods varying from several minutes to an hour. The points on the skin do not correspond to specific nerves, but are designated by a series of longitudinal meridians through which the opposing life forces, Yin and Yang, are said to flow. Although the rationale for determining the meridians is lost in antiquity, the acupuncture points correspond to motor points of the underlying muscles, points at which the motor nerve enters the muscle. It can also be demonstrated that the skin overlying the acupuncture points has a lower impedance to electric current than that of the surrounding skin.

Several aspects of acupuncture analgesia puzzle the Western scientist: (1) that the stimulus does in fact relieve pain through no known pharmacologic action; (2) that the site of stimulation is remote from the site of its pain-relieving action, and (3) that relief outlasts the acupuncture procedure. The pieces of the puzzle of acupuncture analgesia do not fit together satisfactorily. The 'counter-irritation' theory cannot account for the distance between the needle loci and the area at which their effect occurs. *Melzack and Wall's* gate theory is a more attractive hypothesis. It is suggested that somehow the acupuncture needle stimulated the large nerve fibers to close the gate to transmission of painful stimuli. While this theory accounts for analgesia in areas removed from those of stimulation, it does not explain long-term or permanent pain relief.

Recent investigations have tested a possible link between acupuncture and the release of endogenous morphine-like substances (endorphins). Injections of naloxone, a morphine inhibitor, markedly reduce the analgesia produced by acupuncture. However, endorphins would be expected to produce general rather than site-specific analgesia. In addition, endorphin analgesia is very limited temporally and cannot account for the permanent pain relief sometimes achieved through acupuncture.

Much research has aimed to establish or rule out hypnosis as the mechanism behind acupuncture analgesia. Subjective and neurophysiological observations have established that behavior, brain wave activity, and the pattern of analgesia or anesthesia are markedly different in the two states and hypnosis analgesia is unaffected by naloxone. Moreover, it is pointed out that acupuncture analgesia can be accomplished in a larger percentage of the population than the 10 or 15% that can achieve deep trance hypnosis.

Acupuncture has been most commonly and successfully used for treatment of headache, trigeminal neuralgia, arthritis, osteoarthritis, low back pain, cervical spine pain, shoulder pain, and radioculopathy. Properly administered, acupuncture can be repeated with less risk than surgery or pharmacologic treatment. It is, quite obviously, not a generally useful method for patient control of pain and has not, in our experience, played a major role in treatment of the chronic pain syndrome. It holds, perhaps, a firmer place in treatment of patients who have diagnosed chronic pain of the types just enumerated and who have not become enmeshed in the behaviors of chronic sick role occupancy.

6. Surgery

Only a small percentage of patients with chronic pain referred to a pain clinic or a neurosurgeon qualify for surgical intervention. In an informal survey, only 3–15% of the patients with pain other than malignancy referred to comprehensive pain clinics with a neurosurgeon as an active member of the team were treated by invasive types of intervention. Of those treated surgically, only 50–60% obtained satisfactory relief for a reasonable period of follow-up. (Perhaps 90% of patients with pain secondary to malignancy qualified for some sort of procedure.) In contrast, patients referred to neurosurgeons in practice who were not associated with a pain clinic had a 90–95% chance of being operated on.

There is no reason to believe that the make-up of chronic pain patients referred to these two groups is any different. Consequently, *any physician who assumes the responsibility of employing interventions to alleviate intractable pain should likewise assume the responsibility for undertaking the type of extensive patient evaluation described herein,* or some comparable variation.

Regarding those few patients who seem to qualify for procedural intervention, the final decision should not be made until after the patient has completed the behavioral aspects of a chronic pain program and the drug intake is acceptable, that is, narcotic free, or evaluation may be quite misleading. Many patients who initially complain of pain serious enough to warrant surgery or permanent blocks get sufficient relief from a conservative program and do not require invasive procedures. Other patients who seem emotionally stable on first visit later reveal psychiatric evidence of pain behaviors where the surgeon should not attempt any invasive procedure.

Surgical procedures for pain relief in general are of two types – stimulation and ablation. Stimulation procedures function by blocking pain pathways with electrical stimulation or stimulating pathways which inhibit transmission of painful stimuli. They do not ordinarily result in destruction of tissue and are therefore reversible. Transcutaneous stimulation, generally the most useful modality, has already been discussed. Other stimulation procedures involve implantation of a stimulating device. Destructive or ablative procedures interrupt the pain pathway somewhere along its course, depriving the patient of pain and possibly other sensation or emotional response. For the most part, ablative procedures are not reversible. Denervation can result in significant side-effects, the most serious of which are dysesthesia or denervation pain which may be worse than the patient's original pain. There is little place for the use of ablative procedures in the management of chronic pain.

As with any surgery, the decision is reached by assessing the risk:benefit ratio. Nonsurgical techniques carry the least risk, frequently are of significant benefit, and should be considered first. Stimulation techniques ordinarily do not result in permanent alteration of neurological function or present unwarranted risk and, where indicated, might be considered next. Ablative procedures should be reserved for those cases in which, because of the etiology of pain (e.g., cancer), the chance of success is considerable enough to justify the great risk.

Of the stimulation procedures, there is greater risk associated with some than with others, a fact which should be considered in selection of patients for interventions. For example, most patients may be candidates for a trial of transcutaneous stimulation with its minimal risk somewhere along the line. Very few patients, however, have severe enough pain or are sufficiently disabled to justify stereotactic stimulation of deep brain structures.

a) Ablative Procedures

There is little use for ablative procedures in the management of chronic pain! Those few conditions which qualify for ablative procedures involve specific trauma to peripheral nerves or to the nervous system, with well-defined, discretely localized etiology. Generally, the higher in the nervous system a therapeutic lesion is made, the less likelihood there is for permanent pain relief. This may be a function of the increasing complexity and redundancy of pain pathways as the central nervous system ascends toward the brain. Taking this into consideration, a peripheral neurectomy to treat pain of a discrete neuroma might be sanctioned, where it is almost impossible to justify a thalamotomy for diffuse pain of indefinite etiology.

Perhaps the most commonly performed, and least successful, ablative surgical procedure for the treatment of pain of benign origin is dorsal rhizotomy for the treatment of pain resulting from failure of lumbar disc surgery. This would seem like a logical treatment, since theoretically when the surgeon interrupts the offending nerve root, he disconnects the source of the pain from the central nervous system. Unfortunately, this is not so in practice. We do not really know what causes continued radicular pain when decompression of the nerve root fails. Furthermore, we do not know why pain should persist or resume after proximal interruption of the damaged nerve roots. Although there are a number of reports in the literature about successful alleviation of nerve root pain under these circumstances, long-term follow-up reports are sufficiently discouraging to indicate that dorsal rhizotomy should not be employed in the management of chronic pain.

The same can be said of post-herpetic neuralgia. This condition produces severe pain radiating along a single nerve, the dorsal root of which has been invaded by virus, and would seem ideally suited for treatment by interruption of that nerve root. It is felt that the virus invades the next higher neuron in the pathway so that it is present proximal to the point of section. Thankfully, however, 50% of patients with post-herpetic neuralgia demonstrate significant improvement with transcutaneous stimulation. The electrodes can be placed at the site of the pain or across the distribution of the pain, dependent on the response of the patient during trial placement. On the other hand, the production of lesions in the substantia gelatinosa, or dorsal root entry zone (DREZ lesions) may help patients with post-herpetic involvement of individual roots of trunk or limb.

Other ablative procedures are for very specific conditions, such as trigeminal or glossopharyngeal neuralgia, conditions of paroxysmal severe facial or pharyngeal pain secondary to malfunction of those nerves. Although these conditions may persist over a long period of time, they are not chronic pain as defined here. Patients with these conditions generally do not respond well to the comprehensive program described here alone, but require specific therapy directed to the etiology of the acute episodes as well.

There are a number of types of ablative neural block procedures which have been reported repeatedly in the literature, including epidural alcohol, subarachnoid alcohol or phenol blocks, and epidural or subarachnoid iced saline or hypertonic saline injections. Again, these procedures have little place in the management of chronic pain of benign origin. Although initial results are frequently encouraging, long-term results are less so. Despite the simplicity of performing these blocks, they carry significant risks with them, the most serious of which are quadriplegia or paraplegia. Such risks are rarely justified in the face of little chance for long-term pain relief.

b) Stimulation Procedures

The most commonly employed invasive stimulation procedure is that of dorsal cord stimulation or dorsal column stimulation (DCS). An electrode is implanted to lie just behind the spinal cord, usually just outside the dura. The electrode is connected with subcutaneous leads to a radio receiver which is implanted under the skin at a convenient site, usually just under the clavicle or on the side of the abdomen. The patient controls the stimulation by means of a battery-powered radio transmitter about the size of a pack of cigarettes. This transmitter, which can be worn under the clothing or at the belt, is connected by a lead to a small paddle-shaped antenna which is taped to the skin overlying the receiver. Thus, no wires extend through the skin. The implanted portion does not contain a battery, but is powered passively by the radio-frequency energy transmitted through the skin. Dorsal cord stimulation can be employed for pain of the body or lower extremities, since the stimulation must be applied to the spinal cord above the level at which the innervation occurs.

The patient's response to dorsal column stimulation can be tested without subjecting the patient to an operative procedure. Wire electrodes are available which can be inserted percutaneously through a needle to lie in the epidural space and extend through the skin so that they can be connected directly to a stimulator for a trial period. If the patient responds to such stimulation, the wires are designed so that the portion extending through the skin can be cut off and discarded, and a radio receiver can be attached to the portion of the wires remaining implanted, thereby allowing implantation of the electrodes without need of a surgical laminectomy. If desired, however, the percutaneous test leads can be removed, and a dorsal column electrode can be implanted surgically, which requires a laminectomy and suturing of the electrode to the dura. Different neurosurgeons prefer different techniques. In our experience, the stimulation that is obtained with a surgically implanted unit is more reliable than that applied through the percutaneous wire system, if it can be placed in a location to afford sensation to the painful part.

The surgical procedure to implant the dorsal column stimulator is not difficult and requires routine neurosurgical techniques. However, patient selection and evaluation should be extremely meticulous. Consequently, implantation of dorsal column stimulators should be performed only by those neurosurgeons who participate in, or have access to, a comprehensive pain evaluation and treatment program. No patient should be considered for implantation of a stimulator until psychiatric issues are considered and the patient has been evaluated and treated in a comprehensive program setting. Dorsal column stimulation should be used only to supplement a comprehensive pain program in which insufficient pain relief has been obtained. It should not be employed as an isolated treatment modality.

The theory behind dorsal column stimulation is the gate theory of *Melzack and Wall*. Stimulation of the large sensory neurons inhibits transmission of pain. These large sensory neurons entering the spinal cord extend up the dorsal column of the spinal cord, in addition to those collaterals which enter the substantia gelatinosa. When the dorsal columns are stimulated, the impulse travels in a retrograde fashion down the large fibers in the dorsal columns and into the substantia gelatinosa, contributing to the large fiber input of the gate, in hopes that it might close the gate, inhibit the transmission of pain impulses, and afford the patient pain relief.

There is another stimulation procedure which should be mentioned, although it is still too new for its role in the treatment of chronic pain to be accurately assessed, that is, chronic deep brain stimulation.

It was discovered by *Reynolds* and elaborated by *Liebeskind* et al., that stimulation of the periaqueductal gray matter in rats produced pain relief, so-called stimulation-produced analgesia (SPA). It has been documented that stimulation of the periaqueductal gray matter in man or the area just adjacent to the posterior part of the third ventricle produces relief from both chronic and acute pain, although with less demonstrable analgesia than in experimental animals. Such stimulation produced analgesia has been found to be helpful in a small number of very critically selected patients in investigational settings. Its practice should be restricted for the present to those neurosurgeons who are deeply involved in clinical investigation of pain-relieving procedures. Its use should be considered only in the context of a comprehensive pain clinic setting, and only after all else failed to give the patient relief sufficient to minimize disability. It should not be used by the general neurosurgeon and is still considered to be investigational.

The technique involves the insertion of an electrode into the gray matter just lateral to the third ventricle by the use of a stereotactic apparatus. The electrodes are connected to temporary wires which extend through the scalp so stimulation can be employed on a trial basis. If the patient responds, the temporary wires can be removed, and the electrode in the brain can be connected by means of subcutaneous wires to the same type of radio receiver that is employed for dorsal column stimulation.

The effect of deep brain stimulation does not appear to be related to the gate theory, but rather there is some evidence that paraventricular stimulation causes the release of endorphins, the morphine-like substances normally present in the brain. The role of endorphins in the normal state is unclear, but they seem to be related to modifying pain perception, so that an increase in their release may inhibit pain perception and relieve chronic pain or pain of malignancy. Endorphins are chemically related to narcotics, and, interestingly, the effect of chronic brain stimulation can be blocked by the administration of narcotic antagonists such as naloxone. Also as with narcotics, a tolerance develops to prolonged stimulation, so that the patient must be cautioned to employ the stimulator only periodically or its effectiveness will diminish.

Again, such procedures are employed in only an extremely small group of well-selected patients who are not psychiatrically impaired and who have received maximal benefit from a comprehensive program but still have pain of a specific etiology.

Suggested Reading

1   Adams, J.E.; Hosobuchi, Y.; Fields, H.L.: Stimulation of the internal capsule for relief of chronic pain. J. Neurosurg. *41:* 740–744 (1974).
2   Beecher, J.K.: The powerful placebo. J. Am. med. Ass. *159:* 1602–1606 (1955).
3   Beecher, H.K.: Measurement of subjective responses: quantitative effects of drugs (Oxford University Press, New York 1959).
4   Bonica, J.J.: Clinical applications of diagnostic and therapeutic nerve blocks (Thomas, Springfield 1959).
5   Budzynski, T.H.: Biofeedback in the treatment of muscle contraction (tension) headache. Biofeed. Self Regulat. *3:* 409–434 (1978).
6   Budzynski, T.H.; Stoyva, J.M.: An instrument for producing deep muscle relaxation by means of analog information feedback. J. appl. behav. Anal. *2:* 231–237 (1969).
7   Erickson, D.L.: Percutaneous trial of stimulation for patient selection of implantable stimulation devices. J. Neurosurg. *43:* 440–444 (1975).
8   Evan, F.J.: The placebo response in pain reduction; in Bonica, Pain. Advances in neurology, vol. 4, pp. 289–296 (Raven Press, New York 1974).

9 Ferguson, J.E.; Marquis, J.N.; Taylor, C.B.: A script for deep muscle relaxation. Dis. nerv. Syst. *38:* 703–708 (1977).

10 Fordyce, W.E.: Treating chronic pain by contingency management. Adv. Neurol. *4:* 583–589 (1974).

11 Fordyce, W.E.; Fowler, R.S., Jr.; Lehmann, J.F.; Delateur, B.J.; Sand, P.L.; Trieschman, R.B.: Operant conditioning in the treatment of chronic pain. Archs phys. Med. Rehabil. *54:* 399–408 (1973).

12 Halpern, L.M.: Treating pain with drugs. Minn. Med. *57:* 176–184 (1974).

13 Hitchcock, E.R.; Schvarcz, J.R.: Stereotactic trigeminal tractotomy for postherpetic facial pain. J. Neurosurg. *37:* 412–417 (1972).

14 Hosobuchi, Y.; Adams, J.E.; Rutkins, B.: Chronic thalamic stimulation for the control of facial anesthesia dolorosa. Archs Neurol. *29:* 158–161 (1973).

15 Jacobson, E.: Modern treatment of tense patients (Thomas, Springfield 1970).

16 Katz, R.L.; Kao, C.Y.; Spiegel, H.; Katz, G.J.: Pain, acupuncture and hypnosis; in Bonica, Pain. Advances in neurology, vol. 4, pp. 819–827 (Raven Press, New York 1974).

17 Liebeskind, J.C.; Gilubaum, G.; Besson, J.M.; Oliveras, J.L.: Analgesia for electrical stimulation of the periaqueductal gray matter in the cat. Behavioral observations and inhibitory effects on spinal cord interneurons. Brain Res. *50:* 441–446 (1973).

18 Long, D.M.: Cutaneous afferent stimulation for relief of chronic pain. Clin. Neurosurg. *21:* 257–268 (1974).

19 Long, D.M.; Erickson, D.E.: Stimulation of the posterior columns of the spinal cord for relief of intractable pain. Surg. Neurol. *41:* 134–141 (1975).

20 Marquis, J.N.: Relaxation training. Self Management Schools, Inc., 745 Distel Drive, Los Altos, Calif. (1971).

21 Melzack, R.: Psychological concepts and methods for the control of pain; in Bonica, Pain. Advances in neurology, vol. 4, pp. 275–288 (Raven Press, New York 1974).

22 Melzack, R.; Jeans, M.: Acupuncture analgesia, a psychophysiological explanation. Minn. Med. *57:* 161–166 (1974).

23 Melzack, R., Perry, C.: Self-regulation of pain: the use of alpha-feedback and hypnotic training for the control of chronic pain. Expl Neurol. *45:* 452–469 (1975).

24 North, R.B.; Fischell, T.A.; Long, D.M.: Chronic dorsal column stimulation via percutaneously inserted epidural electrodes. Preliminary results in 31 patients. Appl. Neurophysiol. *40:* 184–191 (1978).

25 Orne, M.T.: Pain suppression by hypnosis and related phenomena; in Bonica, Pain. Advances in neurology, vol. 4, pp. 563–572 (Raven Press, New York 1974).

26 Richardson, D.E.; Akil, H.: Pain reduction by electrical brain stimulation in man. I. Acute administration in periaqueductal and periventricular sites. J. Neurosurg. *47:* 178–183 (1977).

27 Roberts, A.H.: Biofeedback techniques: their potential for the control of pain. Minn. Med. *57:* 167–171 (1974).

28 Royal Canadian Air Force Exercise Plans for Physical Fitness (Simon & Schuster, New York 1962).

29 Saletu, B.; Saletu, M.; Brown, M.; Stern, J.; Sletten, I.; Ulett, G.: Hypnoanalgesia and acupuncture analgesia: a neurophysiological reality? Neurophysiobiology *1:* 218–242 (1975).

30 Skinner, B.F.: Beyond freedom and dignity (Knopf, New York 1971).
31 Sternbach, R.A.: Pain patients: traits and treatment (Academic Press, New York 1974).
32 Sweet, W.H.; Wepsic, J.C.: Stimulation of the posterior columns of the spinal cord for pain control: indications, techniques and results. Clin. Neurosurg. *21:* 278–310 (1974).
33 Travell, J.: Myofascial trigger points: clinical view. Adv. Pain Res. *1:* 919–926 (1976).
34 Wooley, S.C.; Blackwell, B.; Winget, C.: A learning theory model of chronic illness behavior. Theory, treatment and research. Psychosom. Med. *40:* 379–396 (1978).

Conclusions

What can the physician do about chronic pain?

Obviously, the best way to deal with chronic pain is to prevent an acute problem from becoming progressive and chronic.

The first line of prevention lies in the accurate management of acute painful conditions, but the practice of medicine is inexact and, in many respects, unscientific. Many conditions defy effective treatment, so that every physician has a number of patients who continue to have pain despite his best efforts.

How does one prevents one's patients from becoming 'Chronic Pain Patients' with all the psychological manifestations and disabilities described herein?

Most important – *talk to your patient*. The reason the patient may not be getting better may have nothing to do with the physical problem, but may relate to the many emotional and social factors discussed herein.

Be attentive to the changes that may take place in the patient's attitude during the course of an illness. It may not be possible to identify a potential pain patient at the initial visit, since the stage may not be fully set. However, reassess the patient's attitude and dependency status repeatedly. A physician all too often develops an initial perception of a patient and then hangs on to it too long.

Beware of pain medications!

All have been designed for the treatment of acute pain, and are inappropriate for the management of chronic pain. Follow the general rule of not beginning any pain medication without a firm plan as to when to discontinue it. As another general rule, analgesics other than aspirin or similar medications should not be used for longer than two weeks, at which time both tolerance and addiction become significant and depression becomes a devastating side-effect.

There is no analgesic for chronic pain!

Recognizing and treating the depression and regression which often accompany chronic illness or disability are important to prevent progression to the chronic pain state. It is difficult for a depressed patient to rally his resources to embark on a satisfactory rehabilitation program, and even more difficult to convince himself that he is recovering from pain. Since depression is a normal sequela of chronic pain and illness, it must be recognized as a separate entity which requires specific management.

Is it always possible to prevent the development of the Chronic Pain Syndrome?

Unfortunately not. Many chronic pain patients are acting out behavior which was developed early in life and for which there is little chance for modification as an adult. Other patients find the chronic pain state to be the most satisfactory adjustment with life – psychologically, socially, or financially – and may have neither the motivation nor direction to abandon their chronic pain behavior. It must be acknowledged that no pain procedure or medication will be any value to such patients, since the perception of pain is only a secondary manifestation of their primary problem.

Aspects of prevention and management of chronic pain are similar. Both, however, require that the physician recognize the development or establishment of the chronic pain syndrome, so the emphasis in management can be shifted from the physician's responsibility to intervene and cure to the patient's responsibility to adopt an attitude that promotes rehabilitation and normal social behavior.

During an acute problem, it is appropriate to advise the patient to restrict activities and to rest. At one point in the patient's program, however, the physician must recognize that enforced rest may be contributing to rather than solving the problem. At that point, a program of remobilization, consistent with the patient's maximal physical abilities, must be adopted.

It is the primary physician who is in the best position to prevent the chronic pain syndrome. The physician who knows the patient and recognizes how the patient deals with illness and distress, and is aware of the interpersonal dynamics of the patient's family, can detect those situations which predispose to the inability to cope with chronic pain. Often the primary physician is in the optimal position to intervene.

Appendix – Anatomy of Pain

It has been emphasized throughout the text that the perception of chronic pain may or may not involve firing of the classical pain pathways, all of which have been experimentally defined in regard to acute pain. However, some basic understanding of the anatomy and physiology of pain perception is helpful to understand the etiology of certain types of pain and the manner in which some specific treatment modalities work, or at least the theory behind the development of them.

Consequently, this brief discussion of the anatomy of pain is provided as an appendix where it is available to the reader, but not at a point where it might detract from the presentation of the major theme.

No attempt has been made to present a complete picture of the pain pathways, which is beyond the scope of this book[1]. However, brief mention has been made of those aspects of pain anatomy and physiology which relate to concepts or treatments discussed elsewhere.

Noxious stimulation causes firing of both small and large nerve fibers which enter the dorsal root. The larger fibers enter as a medial bundle and are dorsomedial to the small fibers. Collaterals of the large fibers go to three different areas.

One collateral ascends in the dorsal columns to the nucleus gracilis or nucleus cuneatus. Here it synapses with second order neurons which decussate and ascend as the medial lemniscus to the ventral posterolateral nucleus of the thalamus. Another synapse is made and the third order neurons project to the primary somatosensory area of the cortex. This dorsal column system ascends to form the lemniscal system to conduct non-painful information and to localize and characterize painful stimuli. It is the most rapidly conducting system to the brain. It is concerned with light touch, proprioception, stereognosis, two-point discrimination and vibratory sensation.

[1] The reader is referred to Willis, W.: The pain system. The neural basis of nociceptive transmission in the mammalian nervous system; in Gildenberg, Pain and headache, vol. 8 (Karger, Basel 1985).

The second collateral of the large fiber that enters the dorsal root synapses at a cell in the dorsal horn of the spinal cord gray matter, which *Melzack and Wall* called the first central transmission (T) cell. The T cells may be the ones to decussate and to ascend in the contralateral anterolateral quadrant of the spinal cord as the lateral spinothalamic tract, the classical pain pathway. Only one-third of these fibers reach the thalamus, but those fibers that do synapse in the same area of the ventral posterolateral nucleus as do the lemniscal fibers. The third order neurons then project to the somatosensory cortex.

The collateral of the large fibers that enter the dorsal root may synapse on the cells of the substantia gelatinosa (SG) to facilitate firing of those cells. When the SG cells fire, they in turn inhibit the synapse of the collateral of the large fiber with the first central transmission cell, presumably by presynaptic inhibition. Thus, when the large neurons fire they cause the SG cells to fire, which in turn inhibit the neurons transmitting pain information.

The small neurons that fire in response to a painful or noxious stimulus may be either A-delta (type III) or C (type IV) fibers. They enter in the lateral area of the dorsal root and divide into two collaterals. One collateral may synapse with the first central transmission (T) cell, as does the larger fiber. The other collateral synapses with the SG cell either directly or through an interneuron. In contrast to the facilitatory effect the large fiber has on the SG cell, however, the small fibers inhibit the activity of the SG cells. Thus, when the small neurons fire, they inhibit the SG cells from inhibiting the pain neurons. The small cell firing allows those cells to fire, impulses are transmitted through the pain pathways to the brain, and pain is perceived.

Many observations cannot be explained by the original theory, and details of the gate have been proven inaccurate. Yet, it is very likely that some sort of gating system works not only in the spinal cord but conceivably at thalamic or subthalamic levels as well. Although the details of the gate may not ultimately conform to the original outline, the general concept has proven to be a useful tool. Indeed, it was the proposal of the gate theory that led in large part to the reawakening of scientific interest in the pain system, an interest which has led to many advances in this area within the last several years.

The gate theory also provided the theoretical basis for a new concept in the treatment of chronic intractable pain; that is, the use of electronic devices to stimulate the large nerve fibers in the skin, in peripheral nerves, or in the dorsal columns of the spinal cord to 'close the gate' in order to relieve chronic intractable pain. Because procedures designed to interrupt the classical pain pathways have been found to be basically unsatisfactory for chronic pain (but useful for pain caused by malignancy), stimulation devices have opened up new possibilities for treatment in a very small well-selected group of patients. Limited success of stimulation procedures appears to be due in part to improper patient selection or failure to address the manifold aspects of the chronic pain problem.

The same multisynaptic pathways may be involved in visceral pain as are involved in slow somatic pain, but the peripheral small nerve fibers may travel with the autonomic nerves which course with the blood vessels. These are probably sensory fibers with their cell bodies in the dorsal root ganglia, even though the peripheral ends run with the sympathetic or para-sympathetic nerves rather than with the somatic nerve. There is no known antidromic mediation of sensation via the sympathetic fibers themselves, but interruption of sympathetic nerves may obliterate pain of visceral or neuropathic origin. The area below the fundus of the stomach and below the corina of the trachea but above the midsigmoid colon, the bladder trigone and the cervix is innervated by the sympathetic nervous system, and pain fibers from these viscera generally travel with the sympathetic nerves in the chest and abdomen. Consequently, interruption of the appropriate sympathetic chain and associated visceral nerves can sometimes alleviate this visceral pain. For instance, sectioning the splanchnic nerves and associated sympathetic chain may alleviate the visceral pain of carcinoma of the pancreas. Interruption of the sympathetic innervation of an extremity may alleviate pain of vascular origin, but it may be because of improvement in blood supply rather than interruption of pain pathways.

A number of ascending sensory pathways have been implicated in the perception of pain. It might be more useful than listing all of these pathways as an anatomical exercise, to consider that the pain-perceiving system theoretically contains three components: the neospinothalamic, the paleospinothalamic, and the archispinothalamic pathways. Each subserves a slightly different function in pain perception and involves somewhat different pathways, although the distinction is not as precise as one would wish.

The pathways are not as clearly defined as presented, some details are simplified here and others are unproven. Nevertheless, one needs a concept to discuss physiologic pain and this concept serves that purpose quite well.

The neospinothalamic pathway has already been outlined. It has few synapses and constitutes the classical lateral spinothalamic tract. This pathway decussates at approximately the same level as the fibers enter the spinal

cord, or within several levels, and then ascends in the contralateral anterolateral quadrant of the spinal cord to the brain. In lower mammals, most of
these fibers terminate in the ventral posterolateral nucleus of the thalamus,
but in man only a few fibers can be traced so far. Those fibers that synapse
in the ventral posterolateral nucleus are somatotopically oriented and synapse with third order neurons which protect to the primary somatosensory
area of the cortex (SI). This pathway is probably involved in the perception
of fast pain, pain that is immediately perceived, sharply defined, and well
localized.

The paleospinothalamic pathway begins primarily as part of the lateral
spinothalamic tract, but concerns those fibers which synapse either in the
reticular formation just below the thalamus or in the intralaminar or centre
median nuclei of the thalamus. The innervation is bilateral by the time it
gets to the brain stem. These fibers synapse with neurons in the diffuse
thalamic projection system, which then go generally to the secondary somatosensory areas of the cortex bilaterally. This pathway may be involved in
the perception of slow pain that is later in onset, burning or aching in
nature, and less well localized.

The archispinothalamic pathway is phylogenetically the oldest and is
the least specific. Fibers ascend in the spinal cord by a multisynaptic pro-
priospinal pathway. It is uncertain whether these neurons surround the gray
matter entirely or, as there is recent evidence, ascend as a relatively com-
pact bundle near the center of the spinal cord. These cells eventually find
their way to the pontine and medullary retricular formation. Further multisynaptic diffuse pathways ascend to the intralaminar areas of the thalamus
and also to the hypothalamus to provide emotional and autonomic
responses to pain. This pathway may be involved with extremely poorly
localized visceral pain. It is recognized that interruption of the neo- and
paleospinothalamic pathways by anterolateral cordotomy is unsuccessful
for the treatment of chronic pain. Frequently the pain, that returns after a
while, is less well localized and aching in nature, may involve relatively
large areas, and theoretically may be transmitted via the archispinothalamic
system. Recent experience suggests that the chronic or visceral pain of
malignancy may be alleviated by interruption of the archispinothalamic
system near the center of the spinal cord, even if the lateral spinothalamic
pathway remains intact.

The areas in the reticular formation and the intralaminar area of the
thalamus to which the paleospinothalamic and archispinothalamic pathways ascend project in turn to the hypothalamus and limbic system. Thus,

pain can affect the hypothalamus and initiate visceral responses of stress and pain. The limbic system provides the affective or emotional response to pain, which partly explains the common occurrence of anxiety and depression with chronic pain.

Thus, we have the concept of pain sensation transmitted via the peripheral nerves to the spinal cord. The initial discrimination takes place at spinal levels through a gating system. The pain information ascends to the brain via several separate systems of progressive complexity. The information is projected to several areas of the thalamus which, in turn, project to other areas of the brain. The sensory discrimination area of the thalamus projects to the primary and secondary somatosensory area, so the individual knows consciously that something hurts, and also the nature and location of the pain. Projection to the more diffuse area of the thalamus and to the hypothalamic and limbic systems lets us know that when we hurt, we feel bad.

Different neurosurgical procedures have been devised to interrupt the pain pathways at different points, and the type of pain relief that results depends on which tract is interrupted. If the neospinothalamic system is interrupted at the lateral spinothalamic tract, pain may be relieved, but the ability to perceive pain is also lost. The patient reports that pain is gone. When stuck with a pin, he reports it as feeling dull rather than sharp. Unfortunately, chronic pain usually returns after several weeks or months, probably mediated by other pathways, even though analgesia to pin prick may persist. Indeed, the change in pain perception itself may become extremely distressing, so-called post-cordotomy dysesthesia.

If the paleospinothalamic pathway is interrupted just below the thalamus or in the intralaminar areas, the patient with chronic pain or pain of malignancy may also report that the pain is gone. However, when tested with a pin, he correctly perceives it as being sharp, but not necessarily distressing. Again, chronic pain usually returns after a time.

If the lesion is in the limbic system, such as in the cingulate gyrus or subfrontal area, the patient may no longer complain of pain. He may look comfortable and no longer require analgesics. However, when asked if he still has pain, he may reply, 'Yes, it is just as intense as it was, but it does not seem to bother me any more'. When tested with a pin, the patient correctly perceives it as being sharp.

It is extremely rare that one need resort to interruption of these systems for the management of chronic pain, although these procedures may be very helpful to manage the pain and suffering associated with cancer.

Subject Index

A-delta nerve fibers 137
Abuse
  alcohol 28
  physical 25
Acetaminophen 104
Activity profile with pain 63, 66
Acupuncture 124–126
Acupuncturists 4
Acute pain 4
  in analgesic development 12
  components of 7, 8
  fast vs. slow 9
  noxious stimulus in 12
  somatic vs. visceral 9
Addiction, drug 42, 95, 96
Agitation
  from narcotic withdrawal 42, 97
  from tranquilizer withdrawal 102
Alcohol abuse 28
Alcohol injections 122, 123, 128, 129
Alpha training 119
Amitriptyline 103
Analgesia
  hypnosis 125
  stimulation-produced 130
Analgesics
  addiction to 96
  for chronic pain 15, 103
  development of 12
  effectiveness of 64
  habituation of 96
  on long-term basis 41, 42
  in pain perception pathway 96
  pain tolerance affected by 42, 96
  potentiating chronic pain 100
  side effects of 96
  sleep patterns with 97
  for symptomatic relief 95
  withdrawal from 96–102
Anemia, iron deficiency 104
Anesthesia areas 73

Anesthetic
  diagnostic 80
  lidocaine and bupivicaine 80, 121, 122
Anger from treatment failures 83
Angina pain 34
Anticholinergic effects of drugs 103
Antidepressants 32
  anticholinergic effects of 93
  for chronic pain 103
  deleterious effects of 95, 96
  for depression of psychogenic pain 93
  for regression 89
  side effects of 93, 103
  for symptomatic relief 95
  withdrawal from 89
Antipsychotic treatment 93
Anxiety
  biofeedback for 106
  heightened body awareness from 33
  limbic system and 140
  from narcotic withdrawal 97
  pain secondary to 33–35, 93
  pain tolerance with 7
  relaxation training for 106
  from tranquilizer withdrawal 102
Archispinothalamic tract 138, 139
Arthritis 104, 126
Aspirin 96
Awareness
  anxiety causing heightened 33
  and pain 31

Back pain
  acupuncture for 126
  cervical 77, 126
  common areas of 77
  distribution of 62
  examination for 78, 79
  as iatrogenic pain 45
  with laminectomy 65
  low 77–79
  trigger points for 79